ISBN: 979-8425201317

This book belongs to:

_____

Introduction

Migraine is a neurological condition that affects about 15% of the population. Headache is only one of the symptoms of migraine. There are other symptoms such as nausea, light sensitivity and vomitting.

This book allows you to track your diet, sleep, stress levels and much more on a daily basis. This makes identifying triggers so much easier and also gives you a record that you can discuss with your doctor.

It's important to write in this book **every day**. Migraines can be triggered by events that happened the previous day. If we have logged our food intake, sleep, etc. it's much easier to identify common triggers, such as:

- Excess stress
- Lack of sleep
- Skipped meal
- Dehydration
- Variable weather
- Storms and humidity
- Alcohol

- Caffeine
- Processed food
- Strong smells
- Aged cheese
- Chocolate
- Skipped magnesium
- Skipped preventative medication

In this book, you can log:

- your meals and snacks
- any medication taken
- your sleep (how much and the quality)
- any exercise you've done
- any relaxation activities
- any stressful events
- the weather and barometric pressure
- how much time outside you've had
- how much screen time you've had
- how much water you've had to drink
- menstrual cycle details
- migraine severity, location and duration
- any other symptoms

Take control of your migraines and get your life back - let's get started!

Date:

Migraine: Y   N

Daily Migraine Log

Sleep:	Time Asleep:	Total Hours:	Notes:
	Time Awake:	Quality: ☆ ☆ ☆ ☆ ☆	

		What I ate and drank	Medicines	How I feel
Breakfast	Time:			
Snack	Time:			
Lunch	Time:			
Snack	Time:			
Dinner	Time:			
Snack	Time:			

Exercise:

Time:	Description:	How I Felt:
Duration:		

Relaxation:

Time:	Description:	How I Felt:
Duration:		

Stress:

Time:	Description:	How I Felt:
Duration:		

Weather:

High Temp:	Atmospheric Pressure:	Notes:

Other:

Time Outside:	Screen Time:	Do you have your period:	Water Drank:

Headache:

0   1   2   3   4   5   6   7   8   9   10

Head Location:

Time Onset:	Duration:
Medication:	Did it Help?:

Notes:

Other Symptoms::

Nausea	☐	Nasal Congestion	☐
Vomiting	☐	Sensitivity to Smell	☐
Sensitivity to Light	☐	Ringing in Ears / Tinnitus	☐
Sensitivity to Noise	☐	Blurred Vision	☐
Neck Pain	☐	Diarrhea	☐
Visual Aura	☐	Confusion	☐

| Date: |
| Migraine: Y N |

Daily Migraine Log

<table>
<tr><td rowspan="2">Sleep:</td><td>Time Asleep:</td><td>Total Hours:</td><td>Notes:</td></tr>
<tr><td>Time Awake:</td><td>Quality:
☆ ☆ ☆ ☆ ☆</td><td></td></tr>
</table>

		What I ate and drank	Medicines	How I feel
Breakfast	Time:			
Snack	Time:			
Lunch	Time:			
Snack	Time:			
Dinner	Time:			
Snack	Time:			

| Exercise: | Time: | Description: | How I Felt: |
| | Duration: | | |

| Relaxation: | Time: | Description: | How I Felt: |
| | Duration: | | |

| Stress: | Time: | Description: | How I Felt: |
| | Duration: | | |

Weather:

High Temp:	Atmospheric Pressure:	Notes:

Other:

Time Outside:	Screen Time:	Do you have your period:	Water Drank:

Headache:

0   1   2   3   4   5   6   7   8   9   10

Notes:

Head Location:

Time Onset:	Duration:
Medication:	Did it Help?:

Other Symptoms::

Nausea	☐	Nasal Congestion	☐
Vomiting	☐	Sensitivity to Smell	☐
Sensitivity to Light	☐	Ringing in Ears / Tinnitus	☐
Sensitivity to Noise	☐	Blurred Vision	☐
Neck Pain	☐	Diarrhea	☐
Visual Aura	☐	Confusion	☐

Daily Migraine Log

Date:

Migraine: Y N

Sleep:	Time Asleep:	Total Hours:	Notes:
	Time Awake:	Quality: ☆ ☆ ☆ ☆ ☆	

		What I ate and drank	Medicines	How I feel
Breakfast	Time:			
Snack	Time:			
Lunch	Time:			
Snack	Time:			
Dinner	Time:			
Snack	Time:			

Exercise:

Time:	Description:	How I Felt:
Duration:		

Relaxation:

Time:	Description:	How I Felt:
Duration:		

Stress:

Time:	Description:	How I Felt:
Duration:		

Weather:

High Temp:	Atmospheric Pressure:	Notes:

Other:

Time Outside:	Screen Time:	Do you have your period:	Water Drank:

Headache:

0 1 2 3 4 5 6 7 8 9 10

Notes:

Head Location:

Time Onset:	Duration:
Medication:	Did it Help?:

Other Symptoms:

Nausea	☐	Nasal Congestion	☐
Vomiting	☐	Sensitivity to Smell	☐
Sensitivity to Light	☐	Ringing in Ears / Tinnitus	☐
Sensitivity to Noise	☐	Blurred Vision	☐
Neck Pain	☐	Diarrhea	☐
Visual Aura	☐	Confusion	☐

Daily Migraine Log

Sleep:	Time Asleep:	Total Hours:	Notes:
	Time Awake:	Quality: ☆ ☆ ☆ ☆ ☆	

		What I ate and drank	Medicines	How I feel
Breakfast	Time:			
Snack	Time:			
Lunch	Time:			
Snack	Time:			
Dinner	Time:			
Snack	Time:			

Exercise:	Time:	Description:	How I Felt:
	Duration:		

Relaxation:	Time:	Description:	How I Felt:
	Duration:		

Stress:	Time:	Description:	How I Felt:
	Duration:		

Weather:	High Temp:	Atmospheric Pressure:	Notes:
	☀ 🌤 ☁ ⛈ 🌦 🌧 🌨		

Other:	Time Outside:	Screen Time:	Do you have your period:	Water Drank:

Headache:	0 1 2 3 4 5 6 7 8 9 10 😀 😐 🙁 😧 😫		Notes:
	Head Location:		
	Time Onset:	Duration:	
	Medication:	Did it Help?:	

Other Symptoms::

Nausea	☐	Nasal Congestion	☐
Vomiting	☐	Sensitivity to Smell	☐
Sensitivity to Light	☐	Ringing in Ears / Tinnitus	☐
Sensitivity to Noise	☐	Blurred Vision	☐
Neck Pain	☐	Diarrhea	☐
Visual Aura	☐	Confusion	☐

Daily Migraine Log

Date:

Migraine: Y   N

Sleep:				
	Time Asleep:	Total Hours:	Notes:	
	Time Awake:	Quality: ☆ ☆ ☆ ☆ ☆		

		What I ate and drank	Medicines	How I feel
Breakfast	Time:			
Snack	Time:			
Lunch	Time:			
Snack	Time:			
Dinner	Time:			
Snack	Time:			

| **Exercise:** | Time: | Description: | How I Felt: |
| | Duration: | | |

| **Relaxation:** | Time: | Description: | How I Felt: |
| | Duration: | | |

| **Stress:** | Time: | Description: | How I Felt: |
| | Duration: | | |

Weather:

High Temp:	Atmospheric Pressure:	Notes:

Other:

Time Outside:	Screen Time:	Do you have your period:	Water Drank:

Headache:

0 1 2 3 4 5 6 7 8 9 10

Notes:

Head Location:

Time Onset:	Duration:
Medication:	Did it Help?:

Other Symptoms::

Nausea	☐	Nasal Congestion	☐
Vomiting	☐	Sensitivity to Smell	☐
Sensitivity to Light	☐	Ringing in Ears / Tinnitus	☐
Sensitivity to Noise	☐	Blurred Vision	☐
Neck Pain	☐	Diarrhea	☐
Visual Aura	☐	Confusion	☐

Date:	
Migraine: Y N	

Daily Migraine Log

Sleep:	Time Asleep:	Total Hours:	Notes:
	Time Awake:	Quality: ☆☆☆☆☆	

		What I ate and drank	Medicines	How I feel
Breakfast	Time:			
Snack	Time:			
Lunch	Time:			
Snack	Time:			
Dinner	Time:			
Snack	Time:			

Exercise:
Time:	Description:	How I Felt:
Duration:		

Relaxation:
Time:	Description:	How I Felt:
Duration:		

Stress:
Time:	Description:	How I Felt:
Duration:		

Weather:
High Temp:	Atmospheric Pressure:	Notes:

Other:
Time Outside:	Screen Time:	Do you have your period:	Water Drank:

Headache:
0 1 2 3 4 5 6 7 8 9 10	Notes:
Head Location:	

Time Onset:	Duration:
Medication:	Did it Help?:

Other Symptoms:
Nausea	☐	Nasal Congestion	☐
Vomiting	☐	Sensitivity to Smell	☐
Sensitivity to Light	☐	Ringing in Ears / Tinnitus	☐
Sensitivity to Noise	☐	Blurred Vision	☐
Neck Pain	☐	Diarrhea	☐
Visual Aura	☐	Confusion	☐

Daily Migraine Log

Sleep:	Time Asleep:	Total Hours:	Notes:
	Time Awake:	Quality: ☆ ☆ ☆ ☆ ☆	

		What I ate and drank	Medicines	How I feel
Breakfast	Time:			
Snack	Time:			
Lunch	Time:			
Snack	Time:			
Dinner	Time:			
Snack	Time:			

Exercise:	Time:	Description:	How I Felt:
	Duration:		

Relaxation:	Time:	Description:	How I Felt:
	Duration:		

Stress:	Time:	Description:	How I Felt:
	Duration:		

Weather:

High Temp:	Atmospheric Pressure:	Notes:

Other:

Time Outside:	Screen Time:	Do you have your period:	Water Drank:

Headache:

0   1   2   3   4   5   6   7   8   9   10

Head Location:

Time Onset:	Duration:
Medication:	Did it Help?:

Notes:

Other Symptoms::

Nausea	☐	Nasal Congestion	☐
Vomiting	☐	Sensitivity to Smell	☐
Sensitivity to Light	☐	Ringing in Ears / Tinnitus	☐
Sensitivity to Noise	☐	Blurred Vision	☐
Neck Pain	☐	Diarrhea	☐
Visual Aura	☐	Confusion	☐

Daily Migraine Log

Date:

Migraine: Y N

Sleep:	Time Asleep:	Total Hours:	Notes:
	Time Awake:	Quality: ☆☆☆☆☆	

		What I ate and drank	Medicines	How I feel
Breakfast	Time:			
Snack	Time:			
Lunch	Time:			
Snack	Time:			
Dinner	Time:			
Snack	Time:			

Exercise:

Time:	Description:	How I Felt:
Duration:		

Relaxation:

Time:	Description:	How I Felt:
Duration:		

Stress:

Time:	Description:	How I Felt:
Duration:		

Weather:

High Temp:	Atmospheric Pressure:	Notes:

Other:

Time Outside:	Screen Time:	Do you have your period:	Water Drank:

Headache:

0 1 2 3 4 5 6 7 8 9 10	Notes:
Head Location:	

Time Onset:	Duration:
Medication:	Did it Help?:

Other Symptoms::

Nausea	☐	Nasal Congestion	☐
Vomiting	☐	Sensitivity to Smell	☐
Sensitivity to Light	☐	Ringing in Ears / Tinnitus	☐
Sensitivity to Noise	☐	Blurred Vision	☐
Neck Pain	☐	Diarrhea	☐
Visual Aura	☐	Confusion	☐

Date:			Daily Migraine Log
Migraine:	Y	N	

Sleep:	Time Asleep:	Total Hours:	Notes:
	Time Awake:	Quality: ☆☆☆☆☆	

		What I ate and drank	Medicines	How I feel
Breakfast	Time:			
Snack	Time:			
Lunch	Time:			
Snack	Time:			
Dinner	Time:			
Snack	Time:			

Exercise:	Time:	Description:	How I Felt:
	Duration:		

Relaxation:	Time:	Description:	How I Felt:
	Duration:		

Stress:	Time:	Description:	How I Felt:
	Duration:		

Weather:	High Temp:	Atmospheric Pressure:	Notes:

Other:	Time Outside:	Screen Time:	Do you have your period:	Water Drank:

Headache:

0 1 2 3 4 5 6 7 8 9 10

Notes:

Head Location:

Time Onset:	Duration:
Medication:	Did it Help?:

Other Symptoms::

Nausea	☐	Nasal Congestion	☐
Vomiting	☐	Sensitivity to Smell	☐
Sensitivity to Light	☐	Ringing in Ears / Tinnitus	☐
Sensitivity to Noise	☐	Blurred Vision	☐
Neck Pain	☐	Diarrhea	☐
Visual Aura	☐	Confusion	☐

Daily Migraine Log

Sleep:	Time Asleep:	Total Hours:	Notes:
	Time Awake:	Quality: ☆☆☆☆☆	

		What I ate and drank	Medicines	How I feel
Breakfast	Time:			
Snack	Time:			
Lunch	Time:			
Snack	Time:			
Dinner	Time:			
Snack	Time:			

Exercise:

Time:	Description:	How I Felt:
Duration:		

Relaxation:

Time:	Description:	How I Felt:
Duration:		

Stress:

Time:	Description:	How I Felt:
Duration:		

Weather:

High Temp:	Atmospheric Pressure:	Notes:

Other:

Time Outside:	Screen Time:	Do you have your period:	Water Drank:

Headache:

0 1 2 3 4 5 6 7 8 9 10	Notes:
Head Location:	
Time Onset:	Duration:	
Medication:	Did it Help?:	

Other Symptoms::

Nausea	☐	Nasal Congestion	☐
Vomiting	☐	Sensitivity to Smell	☐
Sensitivity to Light	☐	Ringing in Ears / Tinnitus	☐
Sensitivity to Noise	☐	Blurred Vision	☐
Neck Pain	☐	Diarrhea	☐
Visual Aura	☐	Confusion	☐

Daily Migraine Log

Sleep:	Time Asleep:	Total Hours:	Notes:
	Time Awake:	Quality: ☆☆☆☆☆	

		What I ate and drank	Medicines	How I feel
Breakfast	Time:			
Snack	Time:			
Lunch	Time:			
Snack	Time:			
Dinner	Time:			
Snack	Time:			

Exercise:	Time:	Description:	How I Felt:
	Duration:		

Relaxation:	Time:	Description:	How I Felt:
	Duration:		

Stress:	Time:	Description:	How I Felt:
	Duration:		

Weather:

High Temp:	Atmospheric Pressure:	Notes:

Other:

Time Outside:	Screen Time:	Do you have your period:	Water Drank:

Headache:

0 1 2 3 4 5 6 7 8 9 10

Notes:

Head Location:

Time Onset:	Duration:
Medication:	Did it Help?:

Other Symptoms::

Nausea	☐	Nasal Congestion	☐
Vomiting	☐	Sensitivity to Smell	☐
Sensitivity to Light	☐	Ringing in Ears / Tinnitus	☐
Sensitivity to Noise	☐	Blurred Vision	☐
Neck Pain	☐	Diarrhea	☐
Visual Aura	☐	Confusion	☐

Date:

Migraine: Y   N

Daily Migraine Log

Sleep:	Time Asleep:	Total Hours:	Notes:
	Time Awake:	Quality: ☆☆☆☆☆	

		What I ate and drank	Medicines	How I feel
Breakfast	Time:			
Snack	Time:			
Lunch	Time:			
Snack	Time:			
Dinner	Time:			
Snack	Time:			

Exercise:	Time:	Description:	How I Felt:
	Duration:		

Relaxation:	Time:	Description:	How I Felt:
	Duration:		

Stress:	Time:	Description:	How I Felt:
	Duration:		

Weather:	High Temp:	Atmospheric Pressure:	Notes:
	☀ ⛅ ☁ ⛈ 🌦 🌧 🌨		

Other:	Time Outside:	Screen Time:	Do you have your period:	Water Drank:

Headache:	0 1 2 3 4 5 6 7 8 9 10 ☺ 😐 🙁 😢 😣	Notes:
	Head Location:	
	Time Onset:	Duration:
	Medication:	Did it Help?:

Other Symptoms::	Nausea ☐	Nasal Congestion ☐
	Vomiting ☐	Sensitivity to Smell ☐
	Sensitivity to Light ☐	Ringing in Ears / Tinnitus ☐
	Sensitivity to Noise ☐	Blurred Vision ☐
	Neck Pain ☐	Diarrhea ☐
	Visual Aura ☐	Confusion ☐

Daily Migraine Log

Sleep:	Time Asleep:	Total Hours:	Notes:
	Time Awake:	Quality: ☆ ☆ ☆ ☆ ☆	

		What I ate and drank	Medicines	How I feel
Breakfast	Time:			
Snack	Time:			
Lunch	Time:			
Snack	Time:			
Dinner	Time:			
Snack	Time:			

Exercise:	Time:	Description:	How I Felt:
	Duration:		

Relaxation:	Time:	Description:	How I Felt:
	Duration:		

Stress:	Time:	Description:	How I Felt:
	Duration:		

Weather:	High Temp:	Atmospheric Pressure:	Notes:

Other:	Time Outside:	Screen Time:	Do you have your period:	Water Drank:

Headache:

0 1 2 3 4 5 6 7 8 9 10

Notes:

Head Location:

Time Onset:	Duration:
Medication:	Did it Help?:

Other Symptoms::

Nausea	☐	Nasal Congestion	☐
Vomiting	☐	Sensitivity to Smell	☐
Sensitivity to Light	☐	Ringing in Ears / Tinnitus	☐
Sensitivity to Noise	☐	Blurred Vision	☐
Neck Pain	☐	Diarrhea	☐
Visual Aura	☐	Confusion	☐

Date:

Migraine: Y   N

Daily Migraine Log

Sleep:	Time Asleep:	Total Hours:	Notes:
	Time Awake:	Quality: ☆ ☆ ☆ ☆ ☆	

		What I ate and drank	Medicines	How I feel
Breakfast	Time:			
Snack	Time:			
Lunch	Time:			
Snack	Time:			
Dinner	Time:			
Snack	Time:			

Exercise:	Time: Duration:	Description:	How I Felt:

Relaxation:	Time: Duration:	Description:	How I Felt:

Stress:	Time: Duration:	Description:	How I Felt:

Weather:	High Temp:	Atmospheric Pressure:	Notes:

Other:	Time Outside:	Screen Time:	Do you have your period:	Water Drank:

Headache:

0 1 2 3 4 5 6 7 8 9 10	Notes:
Head Location:	
Time Onset:	Duration:	
Medication:	Did it Help?:	

Other Symptoms::

Nausea	☐	Nasal Congestion	☐
Vomiting	☐	Sensitivity to Smell	☐
Sensitivity to Light	☐	Ringing in Ears / Tinnitus	☐
Sensitivity to Noise	☐	Blurred Vision	☐
Neck Pain	☐	Diarrhea	☐
Visual Aura	☐	Confusion	☐

Date:

Migraine: Y   N

Daily Migraine Log

Sleep:	Time Asleep:	Total Hours:	Notes:
	Time Awake:	Quality: ☆☆☆☆☆	

		What I ate and drank	Medicines	How I feel
Breakfast	Time:			
Snack	Time:			
Lunch	Time:			
Snack	Time:			
Dinner	Time:			
Snack	Time:			

Exercise:	Time:	Description:	How I Felt:
	Duration:		

Relaxation:	Time:	Description:	How I Felt:
	Duration:		

Stress:	Time:	Description:	How I Felt:
	Duration:		

Weather:

High Temp:	Atmospheric Pressure:	Notes:

Other:

Time Outside:	Screen Time:	Do you have your period:	Water Drank:

Headache:

0 1 2 3 4 5 6 7 8 9 10	Notes:
Head Location:	
Time Onset:	Duration:	
Medication:	Did it Help?:	

Other Symptoms:

Nausea	☐	Nasal Congestion	☐
Vomiting	☐	Sensitivity to Smell	☐
Sensitivity to Light	☐	Ringing in Ears / Tinnitus	☐
Sensitivity to Noise	☐	Blurred Vision	☐
Neck Pain	☐	Diarrhea	☐
Visual Aura	☐	Confusion	☐

Date:	
Migraine:	Y N

Daily Migraine Log

Sleep:	Time Asleep:	Total Hours:	Notes:
	Time Awake:	Quality: ☆ ☆ ☆ ☆ ☆	

		What I ate and drank	Medicines	How I feel
Breakfast	Time:			
Snack	Time:			
Lunch	Time:			
Snack	Time:			
Dinner	Time:			
Snack	Time:			

Exercise:	Time:	Description:	How I Felt:
	Duration:		

Relaxation:	Time:	Description:	How I Felt:
	Duration:		

Stress:	Time:	Description:	How I Felt:
	Duration:		

Weather:	High Temp:	Atmospheric Pressure:	Notes:

Other:	Time Outside:	Screen Time:	Do you have your period:	Water Drank:

Headache:

0	1	2	3	4	5	6	7	8	9	10	Notes:

Head Location:

Time Onset:	Duration:
Medication:	Did it Help?:

Other Symptoms::

Nausea	☐	Nasal Congestion	☐
Vomiting	☐	Sensitivity to Smell	☐
Sensitivity to Light	☐	Ringing in Ears / Tinnitus	☐
Sensitivity to Noise	☐	Blurred Vision	☐
Neck Pain	☐	Diarrhea	☐
Visual Aura	☐	Confusion	☐

Date:

Migraine: Y N

Daily Migraine Log

Sleep:	Time Asleep:	Total Hours:	Notes:
	Time Awake:	Quality: ☆ ☆ ☆ ☆ ☆	

		What I ate and drank	Medicines	How I feel
Breakfast	Time:			
Snack	Time:			
Lunch	Time:			
Snack	Time:			
Dinner	Time:			
Snack	Time:			

Exercise:	Time: Duration:	Description:	How I Felt:

Relaxation:	Time: Duration:	Description:	How I Felt:

Stress:	Time: Duration:	Description:	How I Felt:

Weather:

High Temp:	Atmospheric Pressure:	Notes:

Other:

Time Outside:	Screen Time:	Do you have your period:	Water Drank:

Headache:

0 1 2 3 4 5 6 7 8 9 10	Notes:
Head Location:	
Time Onset:	Duration:	
Medication:	Did it Help?:	

Other Symptoms::

Nausea	☐	Nasal Congestion	☐
Vomiting	☐	Sensitivity to Smell	☐
Sensitivity to Light	☐	Ringing in Ears / Tinnitus	☐
Sensitivity to Noise	☐	Blurred Vision	☐
Neck Pain	☐	Diarrhea	☐
Visual Aura	☐	Confusion	☐

Daily Migraine Log

Date:

Migraine: Y N

Sleep:	Time Asleep:	Total Hours:	Notes:
	Time Awake:	Quality: ☆ ☆ ☆ ☆ ☆	

		What I ate and drank	Medicines	How I feel
Breakfast	Time:			
Snack	Time:			
Lunch	Time:			
Snack	Time:			
Dinner	Time:			
Snack	Time:			

| Exercise: | Time: | Description: | How I Felt: |
| | Duration: | | |

| Relaxation: | Time: | Description: | How I Felt: |
| | Duration: | | |

| Stress: | Time: | Description: | How I Felt: |
| | Duration: | | |

| Weather: | High Temp: | Atmospheric Pressure: | Notes: |
| | ☀ ⛅ ☁ ⛈ 🌧 🌧 🌨 | | |

| Other: | Time Outside: | Screen Time: | Do you have your period: | Water Drank: |

Headache:

| 0 1 2 3 4 5 6 7 8 9 10 | Notes: |
| 😀 😐 🙁 😢 😖 | |

Head Location:

| Time Onset: | Duration: |
| Medication: | Did it Help?: |

Other Symptoms::

Nausea	☐	Nasal Congestion	☐
Vomiting	☐	Sensitivity to Smell	☐
Sensitivity to Light	☐	Ringing in Ears / Tinnitus	☐
Sensitivity to Noise	☐	Blurred Vision	☐
Neck Pain	☐	Diarrhea	☐
Visual Aura	☐	Confusion	☐

Daily Migraine Log

Sleep:	Time Asleep:	Total Hours:	Notes:
	Time Awake:	Quality: ☆ ☆ ☆ ☆ ☆	

		What I ate and drank	Medicines	How I feel
Breakfast	Time:			
Snack	Time:			
Lunch	Time:			
Snack	Time:			
Dinner	Time:			
Snack	Time:			

Exercise:

Time:	Description:	How I Felt:
Duration:		

Relaxation:

Time:	Description:	How I Felt:
Duration:		

Stress:

Time:	Description:	How I Felt:
Duration:		

Weather:

High Temp:	Atmospheric Pressure:	Notes:

Other:

Time Outside:	Screen Time:	Do you have your period:	Water Drank:

Headache:

0 1 2 3 4 5 6 7 8 9 10

Notes:

Head Location:

Time Onset:	Duration:
Medication:	Did it Help?:

Other Symptoms:

Nausea	☐	Nasal Congestion	☐
Vomiting	☐	Sensitivity to Smell	☐
Sensitivity to Light	☐	Ringing in Ears / Tinnitus	☐
Sensitivity to Noise	☐	Blurred Vision	☐
Neck Pain	☐	Diarrhea	☐
Visual Aura	☐	Confusion	☐

Daily Migraine Log

Date:

Migraine: Y   N

Sleep:	Time Asleep:	Total Hours:	Notes:
	Time Awake:	Quality: ☆ ☆ ☆ ☆ ☆	

		What I ate and drank	Medicines	How I feel
Breakfast	Time:			
Snack	Time:			
Lunch	Time:			
Snack	Time:			
Dinner	Time:			
Snack	Time:			

Exercise:	Time:	Description:	How I Felt:
	Duration:		

Relaxation:	Time:	Description:	How I Felt:
	Duration:		

Stress:	Time:	Description:	How I Felt:
	Duration:		

Weather:

High Temp:	Atmospheric Pressure:	Notes:

Other:

Time Outside:	Screen Time:	Do you have your period:	Water Drank:

Headache:

0 1 2 3 4 5 6 7 8 9 10

Head Location:

Time Onset:	Duration:
Medication:	Did it Help?:

Notes:

Other Symptoms:

Nausea	☐	Nasal Congestion	☐
Vomiting	☐	Sensitivity to Smell	☐
Sensitivity to Light	☐	Ringing in Ears / Tinnitus	☐
Sensitivity to Noise	☐	Blurred Vision	☐
Neck Pain	☐	Diarrhea	☐
Visual Aura	☐	Confusion	☐

Date:

Migraine: Y   N

Daily Migraine Log

Sleep:	Time Asleep:	Total Hours:	Notes:
	Time Awake:	Quality: ☆☆☆☆☆	

		What I ate and drank	Medicines	How I feel
Breakfast	Time:			
Snack	Time:			
Lunch	Time:			
Snack	Time:			
Dinner	Time:			
Snack	Time:			

Exercise:	Time: Duration:	Description:	How I Felt:

Relaxation:	Time: Duration:	Description:	How I Felt:

Stress:	Time: Duration:	Description:	How I Felt:

Weather:	High Temp:	Atmospheric Pressure:	Notes:

Other:	Time Outside:	Screen Time:	Do you have your period:	Water Drank:

Headache:

0	1	2	3	4	5	6	7	8	9	10	Notes:

Head Location:

Time Onset:	Duration:
Medication:	Did it Help?:

Other Symptoms::

Nausea	☐	Nasal Congestion	☐
Vomiting	☐	Sensitivity to Smell	☐
Sensitivity to Light	☐	Ringing in Ears / Tinnitus	☐
Sensitivity to Noise	☐	Blurred Vision	☐
Neck Pain	☐	Diarrhea	☐
Visual Aura	☐	Confusion	☐

Date:

Migraine: Y   N

Daily Migraine Log

Sleep:	Time Asleep:	Total Hours:	Notes:
	Time Awake:	Quality: ☆☆☆☆☆	

		What I ate and drank	Medicines	How I feel
Breakfast	Time:			
Snack	Time:			
Lunch	Time:			
Snack	Time:			
Dinner	Time:			
Snack	Time:			

Exercise:	Time:	Description:	How I Felt:
	Duration:		

Relaxation:	Time:	Description:	How I Felt:
	Duration:		

Stress:	Time:	Description:	How I Felt:
	Duration:		

Weather:

High Temp:	Atmospheric Pressure:	Notes:

Other:

Time Outside:	Screen Time:	Do you have your period:	Water Drank:

Headache:

0 1 2 3 4 5 6 7 8 9 10	Notes:
Head Location:	
Time Onset:	Duration:	
Medication:	Did it Help?:	

Other Symptoms::

Nausea	☐	Nasal Congestion	☐
Vomiting	☐	Sensitivity to Smell	☐
Sensitivity to Light	☐	Ringing in Ears / Tinnitus	☐
Sensitivity to Noise	☐	Blurred Vision	☐
Neck Pain	☐	Diarrhea	☐
Visual Aura	☐	Confusion	☐

Daily Migraine Log

Sleep:	Time Asleep:	Total Hours:	Notes:
	Time Awake:	Quality: ☆ ☆ ☆ ☆ ☆	

		What I ate and drank	Medicines	How I feel
Breakfast	Time:			
Snack	Time:			
Lunch	Time:			
Snack	Time:			
Dinner	Time:			
Snack	Time:			

Exercise:

Time:	Description:	How I Felt:
Duration:		

Relaxation:

Time:	Description:	How I Felt:
Duration:		

Stress:

Time:	Description:	How I Felt:
Duration:		

Weather:

High Temp:	Atmospheric Pressure:	Notes:

Other:

Time Outside:	Screen Time:	Do you have your period:	Water Drank:

Headache:

0 1 2 3 4 5 6 7 8 9 10	Notes:

Head Location:

Time Onset:	Duration:
Medication:	Did it Help?:

Other Symptoms::

Nausea	☐	Nasal Congestion	☐
Vomiting	☐	Sensitivity to Smell	☐
Sensitivity to Light	☐	Ringing in Ears / Tinnitus	☐
Sensitivity to Noise	☐	Blurred Vision	☐
Neck Pain	☐	Diarrhea	☐
Visual Aura	☐	Confusion	☐

| Date: | |
| Migraine: | Y N |

Daily Migraine Log

Sleep:	Time Asleep:	Total Hours:	Notes:
	Time Awake:	Quality: ☆☆☆☆☆	

		What I ate and drank	Medicines	How I feel
Breakfast	Time:			
Snack	Time:			
Lunch	Time:			
Snack	Time:			
Dinner	Time:			
Snack	Time:			

Exercise:
| Time: | Description: | How I Felt: |
| Duration: | | |

Relaxation:
| Time: | Description: | How I Felt: |
| Duration: | | |

Stress:
| Time: | Description: | How I Felt: |
| Duration: | | |

Weather:
| High Temp: | Atmospheric Pressure: | Notes: |

Other:
| Time Outside: | Screen Time: | Do you have your period: | Water Drank: |

Headache:

| 0 | 1 | 2 | 3 | 4 | 5 | 6 | 7 | 8 | 9 | 10 | Notes: |

Head Location:

| Time Onset: | Duration: |
| Medication: | Did it Help?: |

Other Symptoms::

Nausea	☐	Nasal Congestion	☐
Vomiting	☐	Sensitivity to Smell	☐
Sensitivity to Light	☐	Ringing in Ears / Tinnitus	☐
Sensitivity to Noise	☐	Blurred Vision	☐
Neck Pain	☐	Diarrhea	☐
Visual Aura	☐	Confusion	☐

Date:	
Migraine:	Y N

Daily Migraine Log

Sleep:	Time Asleep:	Total Hours:	Notes:
	Time Awake:	Quality: ☆ ☆ ☆ ☆ ☆	

		What I ate and drank	Medicines	How I feel
Breakfast	Time:			
Snack	Time:			
Lunch	Time:			
Snack	Time:			
Dinner	Time:			
Snack	Time:			

Exercise:	Time:	Description:	How I Felt:
	Duration:		

Relaxation:	Time:	Description:	How I Felt:
	Duration:		

Stress:	Time:	Description:	How I Felt:
	Duration:		

Weather:

High Temp:	Atmospheric Pressure:	Notes:

Other:

Time Outside:	Screen Time:	Do you have your period:	Water Drank:

Headache:

0   1   2   3   4   5   6   7   8   9   10

Notes:

Head Location:

Time Onset:	Duration:
Medication:	Did it Help?:

Other Symptoms:

Nausea	☐	Nasal Congestion	☐
Vomiting	☐	Sensitivity to Smell	☐
Sensitivity to Light	☐	Ringing in Ears / Tinnitus	☐
Sensitivity to Noise	☐	Blurred Vision	☐
Neck Pain	☐	Diarrhea	☐
Visual Aura	☐	Confusion	☐

Daily Migraine Log

Sleep:				
	Time Asleep:	Total Hours:	Notes:	
	Time Awake:	Quality: ☆☆☆☆☆		

		What I ate and drank	Medicines	How I feel
Breakfast	Time:			
Snack	Time:			
Lunch	Time:			
Snack	Time:			
Dinner	Time:			
Snack	Time:			

Exercise:	Time: Duration:	Description:	How I Felt:
Relaxation:	Time: Duration:	Description:	How I Felt:
Stress:	Time: Duration:	Description:	How I Felt:

Weather:	High Temp:	Atmospheric Pressure:	Notes:

Other:	Time Outside:	Screen Time:	Do you have your period:	Water Drank:

Headache:

0   1   2   3   4   5   6   7   8   9   10

Notes:

Head Location:

Time Onset:	Duration:
Medication:	Did it Help?:

Other Symptoms::

Nausea	☐	Nasal Congestion	☐
Vomiting	☐	Sensitivity to Smell	☐
Sensitivity to Light	☐	Ringing in Ears / Tinnitus	☐
Sensitivity to Noise	☐	Blurred Vision	☐
Neck Pain	☐	Diarrhea	☐
Visual Aura	☐	Confusion	☐

Date:

Migraine: Y N

Daily Migraine Log

Sleep:	Time Asleep:	Total Hours:	Notes:
	Time Awake:	Quality: ☆ ☆ ☆ ☆ ☆	

		What I ate and drank	Medicines	How I feel
Breakfast	Time:			
Snack	Time:			
Lunch	Time:			
Snack	Time:			
Dinner	Time:			
Snack	Time:			

Exercise:

Time:	Description:	How I Felt:
Duration:		

Relaxation:

Time:	Description:	How I Felt:
Duration:		

Stress:

Time:	Description:	How I Felt:
Duration:		

Weather:

High Temp:	Atmospheric Pressure:	Notes:

Other:

Time Outside:	Screen Time:	Do you have your period:	Water Drank:

Headache:

0 1 2 3 4 5 6 7 8 9 10	Notes:

Head Location:

Time Onset:	Duration:
Medication:	Did it Help?:

Other Symptoms::

Nausea	☐	Nasal Congestion	☐
Vomiting	☐	Sensitivity to Smell	☐
Sensitivity to Light	☐	Ringing in Ears / Tinnitus	☐
Sensitivity to Noise	☐	Blurred Vision	☐
Neck Pain	☐	Diarrhea	☐
Visual Aura	☐	Confusion	☐

Date:

Migraine: Y N

Daily Migraine Log

Sleep:	Time Asleep:	Total Hours:	Notes:
	Time Awake:	Quality: ☆☆☆☆☆	

		What I ate and drank	Medicines	How I feel
Breakfast	Time:			
Snack	Time:			
Lunch	Time:			
Snack	Time:			
Dinner	Time:			
Snack	Time:			

Exercise:	Time:	Description:	How I Felt:
	Duration:		

Relaxation:	Time:	Description:	How I Felt:
	Duration:		

Stress:	Time:	Description:	How I Felt:
	Duration:		

Weather:

High Temp:	Atmospheric Pressure:	Notes:

☀ ⛅ ☁ ⛈ 🌦 🌧 🌨

Other:

Time Outside:	Screen Time:	Do you have your period:	Water Drank:

Headache:

0   1   2   3   4   5   6   7   8   9   10
☺   😐   🙁   😰   😫

Notes:

Head Location:

Time Onset:	Duration:
Medication:	Did it Help?:

Other Symptoms:

Nausea	☐	Nasal Congestion	☐
Vomiting	☐	Sensitivity to Smell	☐
Sensitivity to Light	☐	Ringing in Ears / Tinnitus	☐
Sensitivity to Noise	☐	Blurred Vision	☐
Neck Pain	☐	Diarrhea	☐
Visual Aura	☐	Confusion	☐

Daily Migraine Log

Sleep:	Time Asleep:	Total Hours:	Notes:
	Time Awake:	Quality: ☆☆☆☆☆	

		What I ate and drank	Medicines	How I feel
Breakfast	Time:			
Snack	Time:			
Lunch	Time:			
Snack	Time:			
Dinner	Time:			
Snack	Time:			

Exercise:

Time:	Description:	How I Felt:
Duration:		

Relaxation:

Time:	Description:	How I Felt:
Duration:		

Stress:

Time:	Description:	How I Felt:
Duration:		

Weather:

High Temp:	Atmospheric Pressure:	Notes:

Other:

Time Outside:	Screen Time:	Do you have your period:	Water Drank:

Headache:

0 1 2 3 4 5 6 7 8 9 10	Notes:

Head Location:

Time Onset:	Duration:
Medication:	Did it Help?:

Other Symptoms::

Nausea	☐	Nasal Congestion	☐
Vomiting	☐	Sensitivity to Smell	☐
Sensitivity to Light	☐	Ringing in Ears / Tinnitus	☐
Sensitivity to Noise	☐	Blurred Vision	☐
Neck Pain	☐	Diarrhea	☐
Visual Aura	☐	Confusion	☐

Date:	
Migraine:	Y　　　N

Daily Migraine Log

Sleep:	Time Asleep:	Total Hours:	Notes:
	Time Awake:	Quality: ☆☆☆☆☆	

		What I ate and drank	Medicines	How I feel
Breakfast	Time:			
Snack	Time:			
Lunch	Time:			
Snack	Time:			
Dinner	Time:			
Snack	Time:			

Exercise:	Time:	Description:	How I Felt:
	Duration:		

Relaxation:	Time:	Description:	How I Felt:
	Duration:		

Stress:	Time:	Description:	How I Felt:
	Duration:		

Weather:	High Temp:	Atmospheric Pressure:	Notes:
	☀ ⛅ ☁ ⛈ 🌧 🌧 🌨		

Other:	Time Outside:	Screen Time:	Do you have your period:	Water Drank:

Headache:	0 1 2 3 4 5 6 7 8 9 10	Notes:
	Head Location:	
	Time Onset: / Duration:	
	Medication: / Did it Help?:	

Other Symptoms::			
Nausea	☐	Nasal Congestion	☐
Vomiting	☐	Sensitivity to Smell	☐
Sensitivity to Light	☐	Ringing in Ears / Tinnitus	☐
Sensitivity to Noise	☐	Blurred Vision	☐
Neck Pain	☐	Diarrhea	☐
Visual Aura	☐	Confusion	☐

Date:	Daily Migraine Log
Migraine: Y N	

Sleep:	Time Asleep:	Total Hours:	Notes:
	Time Awake:	Quality: ☆☆☆☆☆	

		What I ate and drank	Medicines	How I feel
Breakfast	Time:			
Snack	Time:			
Lunch	Time:			
Snack	Time:			
Dinner	Time:			
Snack	Time:			

Exercise:	Time:	Description:	How I Felt:
	Duration:		

Relaxation:	Time:	Description:	How I Felt:
	Duration:		

Stress:	Time:	Description:	How I Felt:
	Duration:		

Weather:

High Temp:	Atmospheric Pressure:	Notes:

Other:

Time Outside:	Screen Time:	Do you have your period:	Water Drank:

Headache:

0 1 2 3 4 5 6 7 8 9 10	Notes:
Head Location:	
Time Onset: / Duration:	
Medication: / Did it Help?:	

Other Symptoms::

Nausea	☐	Nasal Congestion	☐
Vomiting	☐	Sensitivity to Smell	☐
Sensitivity to Light	☐	Ringing in Ears / Tinnitus	☐
Sensitivity to Noise	☐	Blurred Vision	☐
Neck Pain	☐	Diarrhea	☐
Visual Aura	☐	Confusion	☐

Daily Migraine Log

Date:

Migraine: Y   N

Sleep:	Time Asleep:	Total Hours:	Notes:
	Time Awake:	Quality: ☆☆☆☆☆	

		What I ate and drank	Medicines	How I feel
Breakfast	Time:			
Snack	Time:			
Lunch	Time:			
Snack	Time:			
Dinner	Time:			
Snack	Time:			

Exercise:	Time:	Description:	How I Felt:
	Duration:		

Relaxation:	Time:	Description:	How I Felt:
	Duration:		

Stress:	Time:	Description:	How I Felt:
	Duration:		

Weather:	High Temp:	Atmospheric Pressure:	Notes:

Other:	Time Outside:	Screen Time:	Do you have your period:	Water Drank:

Headache:

0	1	2	3	4	5	6	7	8	9	10	Notes:

Head Location:

Time Onset:	Duration:
Medication:	Did it Help?:

Other Symptoms::

Nausea	☐	Nasal Congestion	☐
Vomiting	☐	Sensitivity to Smell	☐
Sensitivity to Light	☐	Ringing in Ears / Tinnitus	☐
Sensitivity to Noise	☐	Blurred Vision	☐
Neck Pain	☐	Diarrhea	☐
Visual Aura	☐	Confusion	☐

Date:	
Migraine: Y N	

Daily Migraine Log

Sleep:	Time Asleep:	Total Hours:	Notes:
	Time Awake:	Quality: ☆☆☆☆☆	

		What I ate and drank	Medicines	How I feel
Breakfast	Time:			
Snack	Time:			
Lunch	Time:			
Snack	Time:			
Dinner	Time:			
Snack	Time:			

| **Exercise:** | Time: | Description: | How I Felt: |
| | Duration: | | |

| **Relaxation:** | Time: | Description: | How I Felt: |
| | Duration: | | |

| **Stress:** | Time: | Description: | How I Felt: |
| | Duration: | | |

| **Weather:** | High Temp: | Atmospheric Pressure: | Notes: |
| | | | |

| **Other:** | Time Outside: | Screen Time: | Do you have your period: | Water Drank: |

Headache:

0   1   2   3   4   5   6   7   8   9   10

Notes:

Head Location:

| Time Onset: | Duration: |
| Medication: | Did it Help?: |

Other Symptoms::

Nausea	☐	Nasal Congestion	☐
Vomiting	☐	Sensitivity to Smell	☐
Sensitivity to Light	☐	Ringing in Ears / Tinnitus	☐
Sensitivity to Noise	☐	Blurred Vision	☐
Neck Pain	☐	Diarrhea	☐
Visual Aura	☐	Confusion	☐

Date:	
Migraine:	Y N

Daily Migraine Log

Sleep:	Time Asleep:	Total Hours:	Notes:
	Time Awake:	Quality: ☆☆☆☆☆	

		What I ate and drank	Medicines	How I feel
Breakfast	Time:			
Snack	Time:			
Lunch	Time:			
Snack	Time:			
Dinner	Time:			
Snack	Time:			

Exercise:	Time:	Description:	How I Felt:
	Duration:		

Relaxation:	Time:	Description:	How I Felt:
	Duration:		

Stress:	Time:	Description:	How I Felt:
	Duration:		

Weather:	High Temp:	Atmospheric Pressure:	Notes:

Other:	Time Outside:	Screen Time:	Do you have your period:	Water Drank:

Headache:	0 1 2 3 4 5 6 7 8 9 10	Notes:

Head Location:

Time Onset:	Duration:
Medication:	Did it Help?:

Other Symptoms:

Nausea	☐	Nasal Congestion	☐
Vomiting	☐	Sensitivity to Smell	☐
Sensitivity to Light	☐	Ringing in Ears / Tinnitus	☐
Sensitivity to Noise	☐	Blurred Vision	☐
Neck Pain	☐	Diarrhea	☐
Visual Aura	☐	Confusion	☐

Daily Migraine Log

Date:

Migraine: Y   N

Sleep:	Time Asleep:	Total Hours:	Notes:
	Time Awake:	Quality: ☆☆☆☆☆	

		What I ate and drank	Medicines	How I feel
Breakfast	Time:			
Snack	Time:			
Lunch	Time:			
Snack	Time:			
Dinner	Time:			
Snack	Time:			

Exercise:	Time:	Description:	How I Felt:
	Duration:		

Relaxation:	Time:	Description:	How I Felt:
	Duration:		

Stress:	Time:	Description:	How I Felt:
	Duration:		

Weather:	High Temp:	Atmospheric Pressure:	Notes:

Other:	Time Outside:	Screen Time:	Do you have your period:	Water Drank:

Headache:

0   1   2   3   4   5   6   7   8   9   10

Head Location:

Time Onset:	Duration:
Medication:	Did it Help?:

Notes:

Other Symptoms::

Nausea	☐	Nasal Congestion	☐
Vomiting	☐	Sensitivity to Smell	☐
Sensitivity to Light	☐	Ringing in Ears / Tinnitus	☐
Sensitivity to Noise	☐	Blurred Vision	☐
Neck Pain	☐	Diarrhea	☐
Visual Aura	☐	Confusion	☐

Daily Migraine Log

Date:

Migraine: Y   N

Sleep:	Time Asleep:	Total Hours:	Notes:
	Time Awake:	Quality: ☆☆☆☆☆	

		What I ate and drank	Medicines	How I feel
Breakfast	Time:			
Snack	Time:			
Lunch	Time:			
Snack	Time:			
Dinner	Time:			
Snack	Time:			

Exercise:

Time:	Description:	How I Felt:
Duration:		

Relaxation:

Time:	Description:	How I Felt:
Duration:		

Stress:

Time:	Description:	How I Felt:
Duration:		

Weather:

High Temp:	Atmospheric Pressure:	Notes:

Other:

Time Outside:	Screen Time:	Do you have your period:	Water Drank:

Headache:

0 1 2 3 4 5 6 7 8 9 10	Notes:
Head Location:	
Time Onset:	Duration:	
Medication:	Did it Help?:	

Other Symptoms::

Nausea	☐	Nasal Congestion	☐
Vomiting	☐	Sensitivity to Smell	☐
Sensitivity to Light	☐	Ringing in Ears / Tinnitus	☐
Sensitivity to Noise	☐	Blurred Vision	☐
Neck Pain	☐	Diarrhea	☐
Visual Aura	☐	Confusion	☐

Date:

Migraine: Y   N

Daily Migraine Log

Sleep:	Time Asleep:	Total Hours:	Notes:
	Time Awake:	Quality: ☆☆☆☆☆	

		What I ate and drank	Medicines	How I feel
Breakfast	Time:			
Snack	Time:			
Lunch	Time:			
Snack	Time:			
Dinner	Time:			
Snack	Time:			

| **Exercise:** | Time: | Description: | How I Felt: |
| | Duration: | | |

| **Relaxation:** | Time: | Description: | How I Felt: |
| | Duration: | | |

| **Stress:** | Time: | Description: | How I Felt: |
| | Duration: | | |

Weather:

High Temp:	Atmospheric Pressure:	Notes:

Other:

Time Outside:	Screen Time:	Do you have your period:	Water Drank:

Headache:

0 1 2 3 4 5 6 7 8 9 10	Notes:
Head Location:	
Time Onset: Duration:	
Medication: Did it Help?:	

Other Symptoms::

Nausea	☐	Nasal Congestion	☐
Vomiting	☐	Sensitivity to Smell	☐
Sensitivity to Light	☐	Ringing in Ears / Tinnitus	☐
Sensitivity to Noise	☐	Blurred Vision	☐
Neck Pain	☐	Diarrhea	☐
Visual Aura	☐	Confusion	☐

Daily Migraine Log

Sleep:	Time Asleep:	Total Hours:	Notes:
	Time Awake:	Quality: ☆ ☆ ☆ ☆ ☆	

		What I ate and drank	Medicines	How I feel
Breakfast	Time:			
Snack	Time:			
Lunch	Time:			
Snack	Time:			
Dinner	Time:			
Snack	Time:			

Exercise:	Time: Duration:	Description:	How I Felt:
Relaxation:	Time: Duration:	Description:	How I Felt:
Stress:	Time: Duration:	Description:	How I Felt:

Weather:

High Temp:	Atmospheric Pressure:	Notes:

Other:

Time Outside:	Screen Time:	Do you have your period:	Water Drank:

Headache:

0 1 2 3 4 5 6 7 8 9 10	Notes:
Head Location:	
Time Onset: Duration:	
Medication: Did it Help?:	

Other Symptoms::

Nausea	☐	Nasal Congestion	☐
Vomiting	☐	Sensitivity to Smell	☐
Sensitivity to Light	☐	Ringing in Ears / Tinnitus	☐
Sensitivity to Noise	☐	Blurred Vision	☐
Neck Pain	☐	Diarrhea	☐
Visual Aura	☐	Confusion	☐

Daily Migraine Log

Sleep:	Time Asleep:	Total Hours:	Notes:
	Time Awake:	Quality: ☆☆☆☆☆	

		What I ate and drank	Medicines	How I feel
Breakfast	Time:			
Snack	Time:			
Lunch	Time:			
Snack	Time:			
Dinner	Time:			
Snack	Time:			

Exercise:	Time:	Description:	How I Felt:
	Duration:		

Relaxation:	Time:	Description:	How I Felt:
	Duration:		

Stress:	Time:	Description:	How I Felt:
	Duration:		

Weather:

High Temp:	Atmospheric Pressure:	Notes:

Other:

Time Outside:	Screen Time:	Do you have your period:	Water Drank:

Headache:

0   1   2   3   4   5   6   7   8   9   10

Head Location:

Time Onset:	Duration:
Medication:	Did it Help?:

Notes:

Other Symptoms::

Nausea	☐	Nasal Congestion	☐
Vomiting	☐	Sensitivity to Smell	☐
Sensitivity to Light	☐	Ringing in Ears / Tinnitus	☐
Sensitivity to Noise	☐	Blurred Vision	☐
Neck Pain	☐	Diarrhea	☐
Visual Aura	☐	Confusion	☐

Daily Migraine Log

Date:

Migraine: Y   N

Sleep:	Time Asleep:	Total Hours:	Notes:
	Time Awake:	Quality: ☆☆☆☆☆	

		What I ate and drank	Medicines	How I feel
Breakfast	Time:			
Snack	Time:			
Lunch	Time:			
Snack	Time:			
Dinner	Time:			
Snack	Time:			

Exercise:

Time:	Description:	How I Felt:
Duration:		

Relaxation:

Time:	Description:	How I Felt:
Duration:		

Stress:

Time:	Description:	How I Felt:
Duration:		

Weather:

High Temp:	Atmospheric Pressure:	Notes:

Other:

Time Outside:	Screen Time:	Do you have your period:	Water Drank:

Headache:

0 1 2 3 4 5 6 7 8 9 10	Notes:

Head Location:

Time Onset:	Duration:
Medication:	Did it Help?:

Other Symptoms::

Nausea	☐	Nasal Congestion	☐
Vomiting	☐	Sensitivity to Smell	☐
Sensitivity to Light	☐	Ringing in Ears / Tinnitus	☐
Sensitivity to Noise	☐	Blurred Vision	☐
Neck Pain	☐	Diarrhea	☐
Visual Aura	☐	Confusion	☐

Daily Migraine Log

Sleep:	Time Asleep:	Total Hours:	Notes:
	Time Awake:	Quality: ☆☆☆☆☆	

		What I ate and drank	Medicines	How I feel
Breakfast	Time:			
Snack	Time:			
Lunch	Time:			
Snack	Time:			
Dinner	Time:			
Snack	Time:			

Exercise:	Time: Duration:	Description:	How I Felt:

Relaxation:	Time: Duration:	Description:	How I Felt:

Stress:	Time: Duration:	Description:	How I Felt:

Weather:	High Temp:	Atmospheric Pressure:	Notes:

Other:	Time Outside:	Screen Time:	Do you have your period:	Water Drank:

Headache:

0 1 2 3 4 5 6 7 8 9 10	Notes:

Head Location:

Time Onset:	Duration:
Medication:	Did it Help?:

Other Symptoms::

Nausea	☐	Nasal Congestion	☐
Vomiting	☐	Sensitivity to Smell	☐
Sensitivity to Light	☐	Ringing in Ears / Tinnitus	☐
Sensitivity to Noise	☐	Blurred Vision	☐
Neck Pain	☐	Diarrhea	☐
Visual Aura	☐	Confusion	☐

Daily Migraine Log

Sleep:	Time Asleep:	Total Hours:	Notes:
	Time Awake:	Quality: ☆ ☆ ☆ ☆ ☆	

		What I ate and drank	Medicines	How I feel
Breakfast	Time:			
Snack	Time:			
Lunch	Time:			
Snack	Time:			
Dinner	Time:			
Snack	Time:			

Exercise:	Time:	Description:	How I Felt:
	Duration:		

Relaxation:	Time:	Description:	How I Felt:
	Duration:		

Stress:	Time:	Description:	How I Felt:
	Duration:		

Weather:	High Temp:	Atmospheric Pressure:	Notes:

Other:	Time Outside:	Screen Time:	Do you have your period:	Water Drank:

Headache:

0	1	2	3	4	5	6	7	8	9	10	Notes:

Head Location:

Time Onset:	Duration:
Medication:	Did it Help?:

Other Symptoms::

Nausea	☐	Nasal Congestion	☐
Vomiting	☐	Sensitivity to Smell	☐
Sensitivity to Light	☐	Ringing in Ears / Tinnitus	☐
Sensitivity to Noise	☐	Blurred Vision	☐
Neck Pain	☐	Diarrhea	☐
Visual Aura	☐	Confusion	☐

Daily Migraine Log

Sleep:	Time Asleep:	Total Hours:	Notes:
	Time Awake:	Quality: ☆☆☆☆☆	

		What I ate and drank	Medicines	How I feel
Breakfast	Time:			
Snack	Time:			
Lunch	Time:			
Snack	Time:			
Dinner	Time:			
Snack	Time:			

Exercise:	Time:	Description:	How I Felt:
	Duration:		

Relaxation:	Time:	Description:	How I Felt:
	Duration:		

Stress:	Time:	Description:	How I Felt:
	Duration:		

Weather:	High Temp:	Atmospheric Pressure:	Notes:

Other:	Time Outside:	Screen Time:	Do you have your period:	Water Drank:

Headache:

0   1   2   3   4   5   6   7   8   9   10

Head Location:

Time Onset:	Duration:
Medication:	Did it Help?:

Notes:

Other Symptoms::

Nausea	☐	Nasal Congestion	☐
Vomiting	☐	Sensitivity to Smell	☐
Sensitivity to Light	☐	Ringing in Ears / Tinnitus	☐
Sensitivity to Noise	☐	Blurred Vision	☐
Neck Pain	☐	Diarrhea	☐
Visual Aura	☐	Confusion	☐

Daily Migraine Log

Sleep:	Time Asleep:	Total Hours:	Notes:
	Time Awake:	Quality: ☆ ☆ ☆ ☆ ☆	

		What I ate and drank	Medicines	How I feel
Breakfast	Time:			
Snack	Time:			
Lunch	Time:			
Snack	Time:			
Dinner	Time:			
Snack	Time:			

| **Exercise:** | Time:

Duration: | Description: | How I Felt: |

| **Relaxation:** | Time:

Duration: | Description: | How I Felt: |

| **Stress:** | Time:

Duration: | Description: | How I Felt: |

| **Weather:** | High Temp: | Atmospheric Pressure: | Notes: |

| **Other:** | Time Outside: | Screen Time: | Do you have your period: | Water Drank: |

Headache:

| 0 | 1 | 2 | 3 | 4 | 5 | 6 | 7 | 8 | 9 | 10 | Notes: |

Head Location:

| Time Onset: | Duration: |
| Medication: | Did it Help?: |

Other Symptoms::

Nausea	☐	Nasal Congestion	☐
Vomiting	☐	Sensitivity to Smell	☐
Sensitivity to Light	☐	Ringing in Ears / Tinnitus	☐
Sensitivity to Noise	☐	Blurred Vision	☐
Neck Pain	☐	Diarrhea	☐
Visual Aura	☐	Confusion	☐

Date:

Migraine: Y   N

Daily Migraine Log

Sleep:	Time Asleep:	Total Hours:	Notes:
	Time Awake:	Quality: ☆ ☆ ☆ ☆ ☆	

		What I ate and drank	Medicines	How I feel
Breakfast	Time:			
Snack	Time:			
Lunch	Time:			
Snack	Time:			
Dinner	Time:			
Snack	Time:			

Exercise:

Time:	Description:	How I Felt:
Duration:		

Relaxation:

Time:	Description:	How I Felt:
Duration:		

Stress:

Time:	Description:	How I Felt:
Duration:		

Weather:

High Temp:	Atmospheric Pressure:	Notes:

Other:

Time Outside:	Screen Time:	Do you have your period:	Water Drank:

Headache:

0 1 2 3 4 5 6 7 8 9 10	Notes:

Head Location:

Time Onset:	Duration:
Medication:	Did it Help?:

Other Symptoms::

Nausea	☐	Nasal Congestion	☐
Vomiting	☐	Sensitivity to Smell	☐
Sensitivity to Light	☐	Ringing in Ears / Tinnitus	☐
Sensitivity to Noise	☐	Blurred Vision	☐
Neck Pain	☐	Diarrhea	☐
Visual Aura	☐	Confusion	☐

Daily Migraine Log

Date:

Migraine: Y N

Sleep:	Time Asleep:	Total Hours:	Notes:
	Time Awake:	Quality: ☆☆☆☆☆	

		What I ate and drank	Medicines	How I feel
Breakfast	Time:			
Snack	Time:			
Lunch	Time:			
Snack	Time:			
Dinner	Time:			
Snack	Time:			

Exercise:

Time:	Description:	How I Felt:
Duration:		

Relaxation:

Time:	Description:	How I Felt:
Duration:		

Stress:

Time:	Description:	How I Felt:
Duration:		

Weather:

High Temp:	Atmospheric Pressure:	Notes:

Other:

Time Outside:	Screen Time:	Do you have your period:	Water Drank:

Headache:

0   1   2   3   4   5   6   7   8   9   10

Notes:

Head Location:

Time Onset:	Duration:
Medication:	Did it Help?:

Other Symptoms:

Nausea	☐	Nasal Congestion	☐
Vomiting	☐	Sensitivity to Smell	☐
Sensitivity to Light	☐	Ringing in Ears / Tinnitus	☐
Sensitivity to Noise	☐	Blurred Vision	☐
Neck Pain	☐	Diarrhea	☐
Visual Aura	☐	Confusion	☐

Daily Migraine Log

Date:

Migraine: Y   N

Sleep:

			Notes:
	Time Asleep:	Total Hours:	
	Time Awake:	Quality: ☆ ☆ ☆ ☆ ☆	

		What I ate and drank	Medicines	How I feel
Breakfast	Time:			
Snack	Time:			
Lunch	Time:			
Snack	Time:			
Dinner	Time:			
Snack	Time:			

Exercise:	Time:	Description:	How I Felt:
	Duration:		

Relaxation:	Time:	Description:	How I Felt:
	Duration:		

Stress:	Time:	Description:	How I Felt:
	Duration:		

Weather:

High Temp:	Atmospheric Pressure:	Notes:

Other:

Time Outside:	Screen Time:	Do you have your period:	Water Drank:

Headache:

0 1 2 3 4 5 6 7 8 9 10	Notes:
Head Location:	

Time Onset:	Duration:
Medication:	Did it Help?:

Other Symptoms:

Nausea	☐	Nasal Congestion	☐
Vomiting	☐	Sensitivity to Smell	☐
Sensitivity to Light	☐	Ringing in Ears / Tinnitus	☐
Sensitivity to Noise	☐	Blurred Vision	☐
Neck Pain	☐	Diarrhea	☐
Visual Aura	☐	Confusion	☐

Daily Migraine Log

Date:

Migraine: Y   N

Sleep:	Time Asleep:	Total Hours:	Notes:
	Time Awake:	Quality: ☆☆☆☆☆	

		What I ate and drank	Medicines	How I feel
Breakfast	Time:			
Snack	Time:			
Lunch	Time:			
Snack	Time:			
Dinner	Time:			
Snack	Time:			

Exercise:

Time:	Description:	How I Felt:
Duration:		

Relaxation:

Time:	Description:	How I Felt:
Duration:		

Stress:

Time:	Description:	How I Felt:
Duration:		

Weather:

High Temp:	Atmospheric Pressure:	Notes:

Other:

Time Outside:	Screen Time:	Do you have your period:	Water Drank:

Headache:

0 1 2 3 4 5 6 7 8 9 10	Notes:

Head Location:

Time Onset:	Duration:
Medication:	Did it Help?:

Other Symptoms:

Nausea	☐	Nasal Congestion	☐
Vomiting	☐	Sensitivity to Smell	☐
Sensitivity to Light	☐	Ringing in Ears / Tinnitus	☐
Sensitivity to Noise	☐	Blurred Vision	☐
Neck Pain	☐	Diarrhea	☐
Visual Aura	☐	Confusion	☐

Date:

Migraine: Y   N

Daily Migraine Log

Sleep:	Time Asleep:	Total Hours:	Notes:
	Time Awake:	Quality: ☆☆☆☆☆	

		What I ate and drank	Medicines	How I feel
Breakfast	Time:			
Snack	Time:			
Lunch	Time:			
Snack	Time:			
Dinner	Time:			
Snack	Time:			

Exercise:

Time:	Description:	How I Felt:
Duration:		

Relaxation:

Time:	Description:	How I Felt:
Duration:		

Stress:

Time:	Description:	How I Felt:
Duration:		

Weather:

High Temp:	Atmospheric Pressure:	Notes:

Other:

Time Outside:	Screen Time:	Do you have your period:	Water Drank:

Headache:

0   1   2   3   4   5   6   7   8   9   10

Notes:

Head Location:

Time Onset:	Duration:
Medication:	Did it Help?:

Other Symptoms::

Nausea	☐	Nasal Congestion	☐
Vomiting	☐	Sensitivity to Smell	☐
Sensitivity to Light	☐	Ringing in Ears / Tinnitus	☐
Sensitivity to Noise	☐	Blurred Vision	☐
Neck Pain	☐	Diarrhea	☐
Visual Aura	☐	Confusion	☐

Daily Migraine Log

Date:

Migraine: Y   N

Sleep:	Time Asleep:	Total Hours:	Notes:
	Time Awake:	Quality: ☆ ☆ ☆ ☆ ☆	

		What I ate and drank	Medicines	How I feel
Breakfast	Time:			
Snack	Time:			
Lunch	Time:			
Snack	Time:			
Dinner	Time:			
Snack	Time:			

| **Exercise:** | Time: | Description: | How I Felt: |
| | Duration: | | |

| **Relaxation:** | Time: | Description: | How I Felt: |
| | Duration: | | |

| **Stress:** | Time: | Description: | How I Felt: |
| | Duration: | | |

Weather:

| High Temp: | Atmospheric Pressure: | Notes: |

Other:

| Time Outside: | Screen Time: | Do you have your period: | Water Drank: |

Headache:

| 0 1 2 3 4 5 6 7 8 9 10 | Notes: |

| Head Location: |

| Time Onset: | Duration: |

| Medication: | Did it Help?: |

Other Symptoms::

Nausea	☐	Nasal Congestion	☐
Vomiting	☐	Sensitivity to Smell	☐
Sensitivity to Light	☐	Ringing in Ears / Tinnitus	☐
Sensitivity to Noise	☐	Blurred Vision	☐
Neck Pain	☐	Diarrhea	☐
Visual Aura	☐	Confusion	☐

Daily Migraine Log

Date:

Migraine:　Y　　N

Sleep:				Notes:
	Time Asleep:		Total Hours:	
	Time Awake:		Quality: ☆ ☆ ☆ ☆ ☆	

		What I ate and drank	Medicines	How I feel
Breakfast	Time:			
Snack	Time:			
Lunch	Time:			
Snack	Time:			
Dinner	Time:			
Snack	Time:			

Exercise:

Time:	Description:	How I Felt:
Duration:		

Relaxation:

Time:	Description:	How I Felt:
Duration:		

Stress:

Time:	Description:	How I Felt:
Duration:		

Weather:

High Temp:	Atmospheric Pressure:	Notes:

Other:

Time Outside:	Screen Time:	Do you have your period:	Water Drank:

Headache:

0 1 2 3 4 5 6 7 8 9 10	Notes:
Head Location:	

Time Onset:	Duration:
Medication:	Did it Help?:

Other Symptoms::

Nausea	☐	Nasal Congestion	☐
Vomiting	☐	Sensitivity to Smell	☐
Sensitivity to Light	☐	Ringing in Ears / Tinnitus	☐
Sensitivity to Noise	☐	Blurred Vision	☐
Neck Pain	☐	Diarrhea	☐
Visual Aura	☐	Confusion	☐

Date:

Migraine: Y   N

Daily Migraine Log

Sleep:	Time Asleep:	Total Hours:	Notes:
	Time Awake:	Quality: ☆ ☆ ☆ ☆ ☆	

		What I ate and drank	Medicines	How I feel
Breakfast	Time:			
Snack	Time:			
Lunch	Time:			
Snack	Time:			
Dinner	Time:			
Snack	Time:			

Exercise:

Time:	Description:	How I Felt:
Duration:		

Relaxation:

Time:	Description:	How I Felt:
Duration:		

Stress:

Time:	Description:	How I Felt:
Duration:		

Weather:

High Temp:	Atmospheric Pressure:	Notes:

Other:

Time Outside:	Screen Time:	Do you have your period:	Water Drank:

Headache:

0 1 2 3 4 5 6 7 8 9 10	Notes:
Head Location:	

Time Onset:	Duration:
Medication:	Did it Help?:

Other Symptoms::

Nausea	☐	Nasal Congestion	☐
Vomiting	☐	Sensitivity to Smell	☐
Sensitivity to Light	☐	Ringing in Ears / Tinnitus	☐
Sensitivity to Noise	☐	Blurred Vision	☐
Neck Pain	☐	Diarrhea	☐
Visual Aura	☐	Confusion	☐

Date:

Migraine: Y   N

Daily Migraine Log

Sleep:	Time Asleep:	Total Hours:	Notes:
	Time Awake:	Quality: ☆ ☆ ☆ ☆ ☆	

		What I ate and drank	Medicines	How I feel
Breakfast	Time:			
Snack	Time:			
Lunch	Time:			
Snack	Time:			
Dinner	Time:			
Snack	Time:			

Exercise:	Time:	Description:	How I Felt:
	Duration:		

Relaxation:	Time:	Description:	How I Felt:
	Duration:		

Stress:	Time:	Description:	How I Felt:
	Duration:		

Weather:

High Temp:	Atmospheric Pressure:	Notes:

Other:

Time Outside:	Screen Time:	Do you have your period:	Water Drank:

Headache:

0	1	2	3	4	5	6	7	8	9	10	Notes:

Head Location:

Time Onset:	Duration:
Medication:	Did it Help?:

Other Symptoms::

Nausea	☐	Nasal Congestion	☐
Vomiting	☐	Sensitivity to Smell	☐
Sensitivity to Light	☐	Ringing in Ears / Tinnitus	☐
Sensitivity to Noise	☐	Blurred Vision	☐
Neck Pain	☐	Diarrhea	☐
Visual Aura	☐	Confusion	☐

Date:

Migraine: Y   N

Daily Migraine Log

Sleep:	Time Asleep:	Total Hours:	Notes:
	Time Awake:	Quality: ☆ ☆ ☆ ☆ ☆	

		What I ate and drank	Medicines	How I feel
Breakfast	Time:			
Snack	Time:			
Lunch	Time:			
Snack	Time:			
Dinner	Time:			
Snack	Time:			

Exercise:	Time:	Description:	How I Felt:
	Duration:		

Relaxation:	Time:	Description:	How I Felt:
	Duration:		

Stress:	Time:	Description:	How I Felt:
	Duration:		

Weather:

High Temp:	Atmospheric Pressure:	Notes:

Other:

Time Outside:	Screen Time:	Do you have your period:	Water Drank:

Headache:

0 1 2 3 4 5 6 7 8 9 10	Notes:

Head Location:

Time Onset:	Duration:
Medication:	Did it Help?:

Other Symptoms::

Nausea	☐	Nasal Congestion	☐
Vomiting	☐	Sensitivity to Smell	☐
Sensitivity to Light	☐	Ringing in Ears / Tinnitus	☐
Sensitivity to Noise	☐	Blurred Vision	☐
Neck Pain	☐	Diarrhea	☐
Visual Aura	☐	Confusion	☐

Daily Migraine Log

Date:

Migraine: Y   N

Sleep:	Time Asleep:	Total Hours:	Notes:
	Time Awake:	Quality: ☆ ☆ ☆ ☆ ☆	

		What I ate and drank	Medicines	How I feel
Breakfast	Time:			
Snack	Time:			
Lunch	Time:			
Snack	Time:			
Dinner	Time:			
Snack	Time:			

Exercise:	Time: Duration:	Description:	How I Felt:

Relaxation:	Time: Duration:	Description:	How I Felt:

Stress:	Time: Duration:	Description:	How I Felt:

Weather:	High Temp:	Atmospheric Pressure:	Notes:

Other:	Time Outside:	Screen Time:	Do you have your period:	Water Drank:

Headache:

0   1   2   3   4   5   6   7   8   9   10

Notes:

Head Location:

Time Onset:	Duration:
Medication:	Did it Help?:

Other Symptoms::

Nausea	☐	Nasal Congestion	☐
Vomiting	☐	Sensitivity to Smell	☐
Sensitivity to Light	☐	Ringing in Ears / Tinnitus	☐
Sensitivity to Noise	☐	Blurred Vision	☐
Neck Pain	☐	Diarrhea	☐
Visual Aura	☐	Confusion	☐

Date:

Migraine: Y   N

Daily Migraine Log

Sleep:	Time Asleep:	Total Hours:	Notes:
	Time Awake:	Quality: ☆ ☆ ☆ ☆ ☆	

		What I ate and drank	Medicines	How I feel
Breakfast	Time:			
Snack	Time:			
Lunch	Time:			
Snack	Time:			
Dinner	Time:			
Snack	Time:			

Exercise:

Time:	Description:	How I Felt:
Duration:		

Relaxation:

Time:	Description:	How I Felt:
Duration:		

Stress:

Time:	Description:	How I Felt:
Duration:		

Weather:

High Temp:	Atmospheric Pressure:	Notes:

Other:

Time Outside:	Screen Time:	Do you have your period:	Water Drank:

Headache:

0 1 2 3 4 5 6 7 8 9 10	Notes:
Head Location:	
Time Onset:	Duration:	
Medication:	Did it Help?:	

Other Symptoms::

Nausea	☐	Nasal Congestion	☐
Vomiting	☐	Sensitivity to Smell	☐
Sensitivity to Light	☐	Ringing in Ears / Tinnitus	☐
Sensitivity to Noise	☐	Blurred Vision	☐
Neck Pain	☐	Diarrhea	☐
Visual Aura	☐	Confusion	☐

Date:

Migraine:　Y　N

Daily Migraine Log

Sleep:	Time Asleep:	Total Hours:	Notes:
	Time Awake:	Quality: ☆ ☆ ☆ ☆ ☆	

		What I ate and drank	Medicines	How I feel
Breakfast	Time:			
Snack	Time:			
Lunch	Time:			
Snack	Time:			
Dinner	Time:			
Snack	Time:			

Exercise:

Time:	Description:	How I Felt:
Duration:		

Relaxation:

Time:	Description:	How I Felt:
Duration:		

Stress:

Time:	Description:	How I Felt:
Duration:		

Weather:

High Temp:	Atmospheric Pressure:	Notes:

Other:

Time Outside:	Screen Time:	Do you have your period:	Water Drank:

Headache:

0	1	2	3	4	5	6	7	8	9	10	Notes:

Head Location:

Time Onset:	Duration:
Medication:	Did it Help?:

Other Symptoms::

Nausea	☐	Nasal Congestion	☐
Vomiting	☐	Sensitivity to Smell	☐
Sensitivity to Light	☐	Ringing in Ears / Tinnitus	☐
Sensitivity to Noise	☐	Blurred Vision	☐
Neck Pain	☐	Diarrhea	☐
Visual Aura	☐	Confusion	☐

Date:

Migraine: Y   N

Daily Migraine Log

<table>
<tr><td rowspan="2">Sleep:</td><td>Time Asleep:</td><td>Total Hours:</td><td rowspan="2">Notes:</td></tr>
<tr><td>Time Awake:</td><td>Quality:
☆ ☆ ☆ ☆ ☆</td></tr>
</table>

		What I ate and drank	Medicines	How I feel
Breakfast	Time:			
Snack	Time:			
Lunch	Time:			
Snack	Time:			
Dinner	Time:			
Snack	Time:			

Exercise:

Time:	Description:	How I Felt:
Duration:		

Relaxation:

Time:	Description:	How I Felt:
Duration:		

Stress:

Time:	Description:	How I Felt:
Duration:		

Weather:

High Temp:	Atmospheric Pressure:	Notes:

Other:

Time Outside:	Screen Time:	Do you have your period:	Water Drank:

Headache:

0 1 2 3 4 5 6 7 8 9 10

Notes:

Head Location:

Time Onset:	Duration:
Medication:	Did it Help?:

Other Symptoms::

Nausea	☐	Nasal Congestion	☐
Vomiting	☐	Sensitivity to Smell	☐
Sensitivity to Light	☐	Ringing in Ears / Tinnitus	☐
Sensitivity to Noise	☐	Blurred Vision	☐
Neck Pain	☐	Diarrhea	☐
Visual Aura	☐	Confusion	☐

Daily Migraine Log

Date:

Migraine: Y N

Sleep:	Time Asleep:	Total Hours:	Notes:
	Time Awake:	Quality: ☆☆☆☆☆	

		What I ate and drank	Medicines	How I feel
Breakfast	Time:			
Snack	Time:			
Lunch	Time:			
Snack	Time:			
Dinner	Time:			
Snack	Time:			

| Exercise: | Time: | Description: | How I Felt: |
| | Duration: | | |

| Relaxation: | Time: | Description: | How I Felt: |
| | Duration: | | |

| Stress: | Time: | Description: | How I Felt: |
| | Duration: | | |

Weather:

High Temp: | Atmospheric Pressure: | Notes:

Other:

Time Outside: | Screen Time: | Do you have your period: | Water Drank:

Headache:

0 1 2 3 4 5 6 7 8 9 10

Notes:

Head Location:

Time Onset: | Duration:

Medication: | Did it Help?:

Other Symptoms::

Nausea	☐	Nasal Congestion	☐
Vomiting	☐	Sensitivity to Smell	☐
Sensitivity to Light	☐	Ringing in Ears / Tinnitus	☐
Sensitivity to Noise	☐	Blurred Vision	☐
Neck Pain	☐	Diarrhea	☐
Visual Aura	☐	Confusion	☐

Daily Migraine Log

Sleep:	Time Asleep:	Total Hours:	Notes:
	Time Awake:	Quality: ☆ ☆ ☆ ☆ ☆	

		What I ate and drank	Medicines	How I feel
Breakfast	Time:			
Snack	Time:			
Lunch	Time:			
Snack	Time:			
Dinner	Time:			
Snack	Time:			

Exercise:

Time:	Description:	How I Felt:
Duration:		

Relaxation:

Time:	Description:	How I Felt:
Duration:		

Stress:

Time:	Description:	How I Felt:
Duration:		

Weather:

High Temp:	Atmospheric Pressure:	Notes:

Other:

Time Outside:	Screen Time:	Do you have your period:	Water Drank:

Headache:

0   1   2   3   4   5   6   7   8   9   10

Notes:

Head Location:

Time Onset	Duration:
Medication:	Did it Help?:

Other Symptoms::

Nausea	☐	Nasal Congestion	☐
Vomiting	☐	Sensitivity to Smell	☐
Sensitivity to Light	☐	Ringing in Ears / Tinnitus	☐
Sensitivity to Noise	☐	Blurred Vision	☐
Neck Pain	☐	Diarrhea	☐
Visual Aura	☐	Confusion	☐

Date:

Migraine: Y   N

Daily Migraine Log

Sleep:				Notes:
	Time Asleep:	Total Hours:		
	Time Awake:	Quality: ☆☆☆☆☆		

		What I ate and drank	Medicines	How I feel
Breakfast	Time:			
Snack	Time:			
Lunch	Time:			
Snack	Time:			
Dinner	Time:			
Snack	Time:			

Exercise:

Time:	Description:	How I Felt:
Duration:		

Relaxation:

Time:	Description:	How I Felt:
Duration:		

Stress:

Time:	Description:	How I Felt:
Duration:		

Weather:

High Temp:	Atmospheric Pressure:	Notes:

Other:

Time Outside:	Screen Time:	Do you have your period:	Water Drank:

Headache:

0	1	2	3	4	5	6	7	8	9	10	Notes:

Head Location:

Time Onset:	Duration:
Medication:	Did it Help?:

Other Symptoms::

Nausea	☐	Nasal Congestion	☐
Vomiting	☐	Sensitivity to Smell	☐
Sensitivity to Light	☐	Ringing in Ears / Tinnitus	☐
Sensitivity to Noise	☐	Blurred Vision	☐
Neck Pain	☐	Diarrhea	☐
Visual Aura	☐	Confusion	☐

Date:

Migraine: Y   N

Daily Migraine Log

Sleep:	Time Asleep:	Total Hours:	Notes:
	Time Awake:	Quality: ☆ ☆ ☆ ☆ ☆	

		What I ate and drank	Medicines	How I feel
Breakfast	Time:			
Snack	Time:			
Lunch	Time:			
Snack	Time:			
Dinner	Time:			
Snack	Time:			

Exercise:

Time:	Description:	How I Felt:
Duration:		

Relaxation:

Time:	Description:	How I Felt:
Duration:		

Stress:

Time:	Description:	How I Felt:
Duration:		

Weather:

High Temp:	Atmospheric Pressure:	Notes:

Other:

Time Outside:	Screen Time:	Do you have your period:	Water Drank:

Headache:

0 1 2 3 4 5 6 7 8 9 10	Notes:
Head Location:	

Time Onset:	Duration:
Medication:	Did it Help?:

Other Symptoms:

Nausea	☐	Nasal Congestion	☐
Vomiting	☐	Sensitivity to Smell	☐
Sensitivity to Light	☐	Ringing in Ears / Tinnitus	☐
Sensitivity to Noise	☐	Blurred Vision	☐
Neck Pain	☐	Diarrhea	☐
Visual Aura	☐	Confusion	☐

Date:

Migraine: Y   N

Daily Migraine Log

Sleep:	Time Asleep:	Total Hours:	Notes:
	Time Awake:	Quality: ☆ ☆ ☆ ☆ ☆	

		What I ate and drank	Medicines	How I feel
Breakfast	Time:			
Snack	Time:			
Lunch	Time:			
Snack	Time:			
Dinner	Time:			
Snack	Time:			

Exercise:

Time:	Description:	How I Felt:
Duration:		

Relaxation:

Time:	Description:	How I Felt:
Duration:		

Stress:

Time:	Description:	How I Felt:
Duration:		

Weather:

High Temp:	Atmospheric Pressure:	Notes:

Other:

Time Outside:	Screen Time:	Do you have your period:	Water Drank:

Headache:

0   1   2   3   4   5   6   7   8   9   10

Notes:

Head Location:

Time Onset:	Duration:
Medication:	Did it Help?:

Other Symptoms::

Nausea	☐	Nasal Congestion	☐
Vomiting	☐	Sensitivity to Smell	☐
Sensitivity to Light	☐	Ringing in Ears / Tinnitus	☐
Sensitivity to Noise	☐	Blurred Vision	☐
Neck Pain	☐	Diarrhea	☐
Visual Aura	☐	Confusion	☐

		Date:	
		Migraine: Y N	

Daily Migraine Log

Sleep:	Time Asleep:	Total Hours:	Notes:
	Time Awake:	Quality: ☆ ☆ ☆ ☆ ☆	

		What I ate and drank	Medicines	How I feel
Breakfast	Time:			
Snack	Time:			
Lunch	Time:			
Snack	Time:			
Dinner	Time:			
Snack	Time:			

Exercise:	Time:	Description:	How I Felt:
	Duration:		

Relaxation:	Time:	Description:	How I Felt:
	Duration:		

Stress:	Time:	Description:	How I Felt:
	Duration:		

Weather:

High Temp:	Atmospheric Pressure:	Notes:

Other:

Time Outside:	Screen Time:	Do you have your period:	Water Drank:

Headache:

0 1 2 3 4 5 6 7 8 9 10	Notes:

Head Location:	
Time Onset:	Duration:
Medication:	Did it Help?:

Other Symptoms::

Nausea	☐	Nasal Congestion	☐
Vomiting	☐	Sensitivity to Smell	☐
Sensitivity to Light	☐	Ringing in Ears / Tinnitus	☐
Sensitivity to Noise	☐	Blurred Vision	☐
Neck Pain	☐	Diarrhea	☐
Visual Aura	☐	Confusion	☐

Daily Migraine Log

Date:

Migraine: Y N

Sleep:	Time Asleep:	Total Hours:	Notes:
	Time Awake:	Quality: ☆ ☆ ☆ ☆ ☆	

		What I ate and drank	Medicines	How I feel
Breakfast	Time:			
Snack	Time:			
Lunch	Time:			
Snack	Time:			
Dinner	Time:			
Snack	Time:			

| **Exercise:** | Time:

Duration: | Description: | How I Felt: |

Exercise:
- Time:
- Duration:
- Description:
- How I Felt:

Relaxation:
- Time:
- Duration:
- Description:
- How I Felt:

Stress:
- Time:
- Duration:
- Description:
- How I Felt:

Weather:
- High Temp:
- Atmospheric Pressure:
- Notes:

Other:
- Time Outside:
- Screen Time:
- Do you have your period:
- Water Drank:

Headache:

| 0 | 1 | 2 | 3 | 4 | 5 | 6 | 7 | 8 | 9 | 10 | Notes: |

- Head Location:
- Time Onset:
- Duration:
- Medication:
- Did it Help?:

Other Symptoms::

Nausea	☐	Nasal Congestion	☐
Vomiting	☐	Sensitivity to Smell	☐
Sensitivity to Light	☐	Ringing in Ears / Tinnitus	☐
Sensitivity to Noise	☐	Blurred Vision	☐
Neck Pain	☐	Diarrhea	☐
Visual Aura	☐	Confusion	☐

| Date: |
| Migraine: Y   N |

Daily Migraine Log

Sleep:	Time Asleep:	Total Hours:	Notes:
	Time Awake:	Quality: ☆☆☆☆☆	

		What I ate and drank	Medicines	How I feel
Breakfast	Time:			
Snack	Time:			
Lunch	Time:			
Snack	Time:			
Dinner	Time:			
Snack	Time:			

Exercise:	Time:	Description:	How I Felt:
	Duration:		

Relaxation:	Time:	Description:	How I Felt:
	Duration:		

Stress:	Time:	Description:	How I Felt:
	Duration:		

Weather:

High Temp:	Atmospheric Pressure:	Notes:

Other:

Time Outside:	Screen Time:	Do you have your period:	Water Drank:

Headache:

0   1   2   3   4   5   6   7   8   9   10

Notes:

Head Location:

Time Onset:	Duration:
Medication:	Did it Help?:

Other Symptoms::

Nausea	☐	Nasal Congestion	☐
Vomiting	☐	Sensitivity to Smell	☐
Sensitivity to Light	☐	Ringing in Ears / Tinnitus	☐
Sensitivity to Noise	☐	Blurred Vision	☐
Neck Pain	☐	Diarrhea	☐
Visual Aura	☐	Confusion	☐

Daily Migraine Log

Date:

Migraine: Y   N

Sleep:	Time Asleep:	Total Hours:	Notes:
	Time Awake:	Quality: ☆☆☆☆☆	

		What I ate and drank	Medicines	How I feel
Breakfast	Time:			
Snack	Time:			
Lunch	Time:			
Snack	Time:			
Dinner	Time:			
Snack	Time:			

Exercise:	Time:	Description:	How I Felt:
	Duration:		

Relaxation:	Time:	Description:	How I Felt:
	Duration:		

Stress:	Time:	Description:	How I Felt:
	Duration:		

Weather:

High Temp:	Atmospheric Pressure:	Notes:

Other:

Time Outside:	Screen Time:	Do you have your period:	Water Drank:

Headache:

0 1 2 3 4 5 6 7 8 9 10	Notes:

Head Location:	
Time Onset:	Duration:
Medication:	Did it Help?:

Other Symptoms::

Nausea	☐	Nasal Congestion	☐
Vomiting	☐	Sensitivity to Smell	☐
Sensitivity to Light	☐	Ringing in Ears / Tinnitus	☐
Sensitivity to Noise	☐	Blurred Vision	☐
Neck Pain	☐	Diarrhea	☐
Visual Aura	☐	Confusion	☐

Daily Migraine Log

Date:

Migraine: Y   N

Sleep:	Time Asleep:	Total Hours:	Notes:
	Time Awake:	Quality: ☆ ☆ ☆ ☆ ☆	

		What I ate and drank	Medicines	How I feel
Breakfast	Time:			
Snack	Time:			
Lunch	Time:			
Snack	Time:			
Dinner	Time:			
Snack	Time:			

Exercise:	Time:	Description:	How I Felt:
	Duration:		

Relaxation:	Time:	Description:	How I Felt:
	Duration:		

Stress:	Time:	Description:	How I Felt:
	Duration:		

Weather:

High Temp:	Atmospheric Pressure:	Notes:

Other:

Time Outside:	Screen Time:	Do you have your period:	Water Drank:

Headache:

0 1 2 3 4 5 6 7 8 9 10	Notes:
Head Location:	
Time Onset: / Duration:	
Medication: / Did it Help?:	

Other Symptoms::

Nausea	☐	Nasal Congestion	☐
Vomiting	☐	Sensitivity to Smell	☐
Sensitivity to Light	☐	Ringing in Ears / Tinnitus	☐
Sensitivity to Noise	☐	Blurred Vision	☐
Neck Pain	☐	Diarrhea	☐
Visual Aura	☐	Confusion	☐

Date:

Migraine:　　Y　　N

Daily Migraine Log

Sleep:	Time Asleep:	Total Hours:	Notes:
	Time Awake:	Quality: ☆ ☆ ☆ ☆ ☆	

		What I ate and drank	Medicines	How I feel
Breakfast	Time:			
Snack	Time:			
Lunch	Time:			
Snack	Time:			
Dinner	Time:			
Snack	Time:			

Exercise:

Time:	Description:	How I Felt:
Duration:		

Relaxation:

Time:	Description:	How I Felt:
Duration:		

Stress:

Time:	Description:	How I Felt:
Duration:		

Weather:

High Temp:	Atmospheric Pressure:	Notes:

Other:

Time Outside:	Screen Time:	Do you have your period:	Water Drank:

Headache:

0   1   2   3   4   5   6   7   8   9   10

Notes:

Head Location:

Time Onset:	Duration:
Medication:	Did it Help?:

Other Symptoms::

Nausea	☐	Nasal Congestion	☐
Vomiting	☐	Sensitivity to Smell	☐
Sensitivity to Light	☐	Ringing in Ears / Tinnitus	☐
Sensitivity to Noise	☐	Blurred Vision	☐
Neck Pain	☐	Diarrhea	☐
Visual Aura	☐	Confusion	☐

Date:

Migraine: Y N

Daily Migraine Log

Sleep:	Time Asleep:	Total Hours:	Notes:
	Time Awake:	Quality: ☆☆☆☆☆	

		What I ate and drank	Medicines	How I feel
Breakfast	Time:			
Snack	Time:			
Lunch	Time:			
Snack	Time:			
Dinner	Time:			
Snack	Time:			

Exercise:

Time:	Description:	How I Felt:
Duration:		

Relaxation:

Time:	Description:	How I Felt:
Duration:		

Stress:

Time:	Description:	How I Felt:
Duration:		

Weather:

High Temp:	Atmospheric Pressure:	Notes:

Other:

Time Outside:	Screen Time:	Do you have your period:	Water Drank:

Headache:

0   1   2   3   4   5   6   7   8   9   10   Notes:

Head Location:

Time Onset:	Duration:
Medication:	Did it Help?:

Other Symptoms::

Nausea	☐	Nasal Congestion	☐
Vomiting	☐	Sensitivity to Smell	☐
Sensitivity to Light	☐	Ringing in Ears / Tinnitus	☐
Sensitivity to Noise	☐	Blurred Vision	☐
Neck Pain	☐	Diarrhea	☐
Visual Aura	☐	Confusion	☐

Date:	
Migraine: Y N	# Daily Migraine Log

Sleep:

	Time Asleep:	Total Hours:	Notes:
	Time Awake:	Quality: ☆ ☆ ☆ ☆ ☆	

		What I ate and drank	Medicines	How I feel
Breakfast	Time:			
Snack	Time:			
Lunch	Time:			
Snack	Time:			
Dinner	Time:			
Snack	Time:			

| **Exercise:** | Time:
 Duration: | Description: | How I Felt: |

Exercise:
- Time:
- Duration:
- Description:
- How I Felt:

Relaxation:
- Time:
- Duration:
- Description:
- How I Felt:

Stress:
- Time:
- Duration:
- Description:
- How I Felt:

Weather:
- High Temp:
- Atmospheric Pressure:
- Notes:

Other:
- Time Outside:
- Screen Time:
- Do you have your period:
- Water Drank:

Headache:

0   1   2   3   4   5   6   7   8   9   10

Notes:

Head Location:

- Time Onset:
- Duration:
- Medication:
- Did it Help?:

Other Symptoms::

Nausea	☐		Nasal Congestion	☐
Vomiting	☐		Sensitivity to Smell	☐
Sensitivity to Light	☐		Ringing in Ears / Tinnitus	☐
Sensitivity to Noise	☐		Blurred Vision	☐
Neck Pain	☐		Diarrhea	☐
Visual Aura	☐		Confusion	☐

Date:

Migraine: Y   N

Daily Migraine Log

Sleep:	Time Asleep:	Total Hours:	Notes:
	Time Awake:	Quality: ☆ ☆ ☆ ☆ ☆	

		What I ate and drank	Medicines	How I feel
Breakfast	Time:			
Snack	Time:			
Lunch	Time:			
Snack	Time:			
Dinner	Time:			
Snack	Time:			

Exercise:

Time:	Description:	How I Felt:
Duration:		

Relaxation:

Time:	Description:	How I Felt:
Duration:		

Stress:

Time:	Description:	How I Felt:
Duration:		

Weather:

High Temp:	Atmospheric Pressure:	Notes:

Other:

Time Outside:	Screen Time:	Do you have your period:	Water Drank:

Headache:

0 1 2 3 4 5 6 7 8 9 10

Notes:

Head Location:

Time Onset:	Duration:
Medication:	Did it Help?:

Other Symptoms::

Nausea	☐	Nasal Congestion	☐
Vomiting	☐	Sensitivity to Smell	☐
Sensitivity to Light	☐	Ringing in Ears / Tinnitus	☐
Sensitivity to Noise	☐	Blurred Vision	☐
Neck Pain	☐	Diarrhea	☐
Visual Aura	☐	Confusion	☐

Daily Migraine Log

Date:

Migraine: Y   N

Sleep:			
Time Asleep:	Total Hours:	Notes:	
Time Awake:	Quality: ☆☆☆☆☆		

		What I ate and drank	Medicines	How I feel
Breakfast	Time:			
Snack	Time:			
Lunch	Time:			
Snack	Time:			
Dinner	Time:			
Snack	Time:			

| **Exercise:** | Time: | Description: | How I Felt: |
| | Duration: | | |

| **Relaxation:** | Time: | Description: | How I Felt: |
| | Duration: | | |

| **Stress:** | Time: | Description: | How I Felt: |
| | Duration: | | |

Weather:

| High Temp: | Atmospheric Pressure: | Notes: |

Other:

| Time Outside: | Screen Time: | Do you have your period: | Water Drank: |

Headache:

| 0 1 2 3 4 5 6 7 8 9 10 | Notes: |

| Head Location: |
| Time Onset: | Duration: |
| Medication: | Did it Help?: |

Other Symptoms:

Nausea	☐	Nasal Congestion	☐
Vomiting	☐	Sensitivity to Smell	☐
Sensitivity to Light	☐	Ringing in Ears / Tinnitus	☐
Sensitivity to Noise	☐	Blurred Vision	☐
Neck Pain	☐	Diarrhea	☐
Visual Aura	☐	Confusion	☐

Date:

Migraine: Y   N

Daily Migraine Log

Sleep:	Time Asleep:	Total Hours:	Notes:
	Time Awake:	Quality: ☆☆☆☆☆	

		What I ate and drank	Medicines	How I feel
Breakfast	Time:			
Snack	Time:			
Lunch	Time:			
Snack	Time:			
Dinner	Time:			
Snack	Time:			

| **Exercise:** | Time: | Description: | How I Felt: |
| | Duration: | | |

| **Relaxation:** | Time: | Description: | How I Felt: |
| | Duration: | | |

| **Stress:** | Time: | Description: | How I Felt: |
| | Duration: | | |

| **Weather:** | High Temp: | Atmospheric Pressure: | Notes: |

| **Other:** | Time Outside: | Screen Time: | Do you have your period: | Water Drank: |

Headache:

0	1	2	3	4	5	6	7	8	9	10	Notes:

Head Location:

| Time Onset: | Duration: |
| Medication: | Did it Help?: |

Other Symptoms::

Nausea	☐	Nasal Congestion	☐
Vomiting	☐	Sensitivity to Smell	☐
Sensitivity to Light	☐	Ringing in Ears / Tinnitus	☐
Sensitivity to Noise	☐	Blurred Vision	☐
Neck Pain	☐	Diarrhea	☐
Visual Aura	☐	Confusion	☐

Daily Migraine Log

Date:

Migraine:　　Y　　N

Sleep:	Time Asleep:	Total Hours:	Notes:
	Time Awake:	Quality: ☆☆☆☆☆	

		What I ate and drank	Medicines	How I feel
Breakfast	Time:			
Snack	Time:			
Lunch	Time:			
Snack	Time:			
Dinner	Time:			
Snack	Time:			

Exercise:	Time:	Description:	How I Felt:
	Duration:		

Relaxation:	Time:	Description:	How I Felt:
	Duration:		

Stress:	Time:	Description:	How I Felt:
	Duration:		

Weather:

High Temp:	Atmospheric Pressure:	Notes:

Other:

Time Outside:	Screen Time:	Do you have your period:	Water Drank:

Headache:

0 1 2 3 4 5 6 7 8 9 10	Notes:

Head Location:

Time Onset:	Duration:
Medication:	Did it Help?:

Other Symptoms::

Nausea	☐	Nasal Congestion	☐
Vomiting	☐	Sensitivity to Smell	☐
Sensitivity to Light	☐	Ringing in Ears / Tinnitus	☐
Sensitivity to Noise	☐	Blurred Vision	☐
Neck Pain	☐	Diarrhea	☐
Visual Aura	☐	Confusion	☐

Date:

Migraine: Y   N

Daily Migraine Log

Sleep:	Time Asleep:	Total Hours:	Notes:
	Time Awake:	Quality: ☆ ☆ ☆ ☆ ☆	

		What I ate and drank	Medicines	How I feel
Breakfast	Time:			
Snack	Time:			
Lunch	Time:			
Snack	Time:			
Dinner	Time:			
Snack	Time:			

Exercise:

Time:	Description:	How I Felt:
Duration:		

Relaxation:

Time:	Description:	How I Felt:
Duration:		

Stress:

Time:	Description:	How I Felt:
Duration:		

Weather:

High Temp:	Atmospheric Pressure:	Notes:

Other:

Time Outside:	Screen Time:	Do you have your period:	Water Drank:

Headache:

0 1 2 3 4 5 6 7 8 9 10	Notes:
Head Location:	
Time Onset:	Duration:
Medication:	Did it Help?:

Other Symptoms::

Nausea	☐	Nasal Congestion	☐
Vomiting	☐	Sensitivity to Smell	☐
Sensitivity to Light	☐	Ringing in Ears / Tinnitus	☐
Sensitivity to Noise	☐	Blurred Vision	☐
Neck Pain	☐	Diarrhea	☐
Visual Aura	☐	Confusion	☐

| Date: |
| Migraine: Y N |

Daily Migraine Log

	Time Asleep:	Total Hours:	Notes:
Sleep:	Time Awake:	Quality: ☆☆☆☆☆	

		What I ate and drank	Medicines	How I feel
Breakfast	Time:			
Snack	Time:			
Lunch	Time:			
Snack	Time:			
Dinner	Time:			
Snack	Time:			

Exercise:

Time:	Description:	How I Felt:
Duration:		

Relaxation:

Time:	Description:	How I Felt:
Duration:		

Stress:

Time:	Description:	How I Felt:
Duration:		

Weather:

High Temp:	Atmospheric Pressure:	Notes:

Other:

Time Outside:	Screen Time:	Do you have your period:	Water Drank:

Headache:

0	1	2	3	4	5	6	7	8	9	10	Notes:

Head Location:

Time Onset:	Duration:
Medication:	Did it Help?:

Other Symptoms::

Nausea	☐	Nasal Congestion	☐
Vomiting	☐	Sensitivity to Smell	☐
Sensitivity to Light	☐	Ringing in Ears / Tinnitus	☐
Sensitivity to Noise	☐	Blurred Vision	☐
Neck Pain	☐	Diarrhea	☐
Visual Aura	☐	Confusion	☐

Date:

Migraine: Y   N

Daily Migraine Log

Sleep:	Time Asleep:	Total Hours:	Notes:
	Time Awake:	Quality: ☆ ☆ ☆ ☆ ☆	

		What I ate and drank	Medicines	How I feel
Breakfast	Time:			
Snack	Time:			
Lunch	Time:			
Snack	Time:			
Dinner	Time:			
Snack	Time:			

Exercise:	Time: Duration:	Description:	How I Felt:
Relaxation:	Time: Duration:	Description:	How I Felt:
Stress:	Time: Duration:	Description:	How I Felt:

Weather:	High Temp:	Atmospheric Pressure:	Notes:

Other:	Time Outside:	Screen Time:	Do you have your period:	Water Drank:

Headache:

0	1	2	3	4	5	6	7	8	9	10	Notes:

Head Location:

Time Onset:	Duration:
Medication:	Did it Help?:

Other Symptoms::

Nausea	☐	Nasal Congestion	☐
Vomiting	☐	Sensitivity to Smell	☐
Sensitivity to Light	☐	Ringing in Ears / Tinnitus	☐
Sensitivity to Noise	☐	Blurred Vision	☐
Neck Pain	☐	Diarrhea	☐
Visual Aura	☐	Confusion	☐

Date:

Migraine: Y   N

Daily Migraine Log

Sleep:	Time Asleep:	Total Hours:	Notes:
	Time Awake:	Quality: ☆ ☆ ☆ ☆ ☆	

		What I ate and drank	Medicines	How I feel
Breakfast	Time:			
Snack	Time:			
Lunch	Time:			
Snack	Time:			
Dinner	Time:			
Snack	Time:			

Exercise:

Time:	Description:	How I Felt:
Duration:		

Relaxation:

Time:	Description:	How I Felt:
Duration:		

Stress:

Time:	Description:	How I Felt:
Duration:		

Weather:

High Temp:	Atmospheric Pressure:	Notes:

Other:

Time Outside:	Screen Time:	Do you have your period:	Water Drank:

Headache:

0 1 2 3 4 5 6 7 8 9 10	Notes:

Head Location:

Time Onset:	Duration:
Medication:	Did it Help?:

Other Symptoms::

Nausea	☐	Nasal Congestion	☐
Vomiting	☐	Sensitivity to Smell	☐
Sensitivity to Light	☐	Ringing in Ears / Tinnitus	☐
Sensitivity to Noise	☐	Blurred Vision	☐
Neck Pain	☐	Diarrhea	☐
Visual Aura	☐	Confusion	☐

| Date: |
| Migraine: Y   N |

Daily Migraine Log

Sleep:	Time Asleep:	Total Hours:	Notes:
	Time Awake:	Quality: ☆ ☆ ☆ ☆ ☆	

		What I ate and drank	Medicines	How I feel
Breakfast	Time:			
Snack	Time:			
Lunch	Time:			
Snack	Time:			
Dinner	Time:			
Snack	Time:			

Exercise:

Time:	Description:	How I Felt:
Duration:		

Relaxation:

Time:	Description:	How I Felt:
Duration:		

Stress:

Time:	Description:	How I Felt:
Duration:		

Weather:

High Temp:	Atmospheric Pressure:	Notes:

Other:

Time Outside:	Screen Time:	Do you have your period:	Water Drank:

Headache:

0   1   2   3   4   5   6   7   8   9   10

Notes:

Head Location:

Time Onset:	Duration:
Medication:	Did it Help?:

Other Symptoms::

Nausea	☐	Nasal Congestion	☐
Vomiting	☐	Sensitivity to Smell	☐
Sensitivity to Light	☐	Ringing in Ears / Tinnitus	☐
Sensitivity to Noise	☐	Blurred Vision	☐
Neck Pain	☐	Diarrhea	☐
Visual Aura	☐	Confusion	☐

Date:

Migraine: Y   N

Daily Migraine Log

Sleep:	Time Asleep:	Total Hours:	Notes:
	Time Awake:	Quality: ☆ ☆ ☆ ☆ ☆	

		What I ate and drank	Medicines	How I feel
Breakfast	Time:			
Snack	Time:			
Lunch	Time:			
Snack	Time:			
Dinner	Time:			
Snack	Time:			

Exercise:	Time: Duration:	Description:	How I Felt:

Relaxation:	Time: Duration:	Description:	How I Felt:

Stress:	Time: Duration:	Description:	How I Felt:

Weather:

High Temp:	Atmospheric Pressure:	Notes:

Other:

Time Outside:	Screen Time:	Do you have your period:	Water Drank:

Headache:

0 1 2 3 4 5 6 7 8 9 10	Notes:
Head Location:	

Time Onset:	Duration:
Medication:	Did it Help?:

Other Symptoms::

Nausea	☐	Nasal Congestion	☐
Vomiting	☐	Sensitivity to Smell	☐
Sensitivity to Light	☐	Ringing in Ears / Tinnitus	☐
Sensitivity to Noise	☐	Blurred Vision	☐
Neck Pain	☐	Diarrhea	☐
Visual Aura	☐	Confusion	☐

Date:

Migraine: Y   N

Daily Migraine Log

Sleep:	Time Asleep:	Total Hours:	Notes:
	Time Awake:	Quality: ☆ ☆ ☆ ☆ ☆	

		What I ate and drank	Medicines	How I feel
Breakfast	Time:			
Snack	Time:			
Lunch	Time:			
Snack	Time:			
Dinner	Time:			
Snack	Time:			

Exercise:	Time:	Description:	How I Felt:
	Duration:		

Relaxation:	Time:	Description:	How I Felt:
	Duration:		

Stress:	Time:	Description:	How I Felt:
	Duration:		

Weather:	High Temp:	Atmospheric Pressure:	Notes:

Other:	Time Outside:	Screen Time:	Do you have your period:	Water Drank:

Headache:

0 1 2 3 4 5 6 7 8 9 10	Notes:
Head Location:	
Time Onset:	Duration:	
Medication:	Did it Help?:	

Other Symptoms::

Nausea	☐	Nasal Congestion	☐
Vomiting	☐	Sensitivity to Smell	☐
Sensitivity to Light	☐	Ringing in Ears / Tinnitus	☐
Sensitivity to Noise	☐	Blurred Vision	☐
Neck Pain	☐	Diarrhea	☐
Visual Aura	☐	Confusion	☐

| Date: |
| Migraine: Y   N |

Daily Migraine Log

Sleep:	Time Asleep:	Total Hours:	Notes:	
	Time Awake:	Quality: ☆ ☆ ☆ ☆ ☆		

		What I ate and drank	Medicines	How I feel
Breakfast	Time:			
Snack	Time:			
Lunch	Time:			
Snack	Time:			
Dinner	Time:			
Snack	Time:			

Exercise:

Time:	Description:	How I Felt:
Duration:		

Relaxation:

Time:	Description:	How I Felt:
Duration:		

Stress:

Time:	Description:	How I Felt:
Duration:		

Weather:

High Temp:	Atmospheric Pressure:	Notes:

Other:

Time Outside:	Screen Time:	Do you have your period:	Water Drank:

Headache:

0   1   2   3   4   5   6   7   8   9   10

Notes:

Head Location:

Time Onset:	Duration:
Medication:	Did it Help?:

Other Symptoms::

Nausea	☐	Nasal Congestion	☐
Vomiting	☐	Sensitivity to Smell	☐
Sensitivity to Light	☐	Ringing in Ears / Tinnitus	☐
Sensitivity to Noise	☐	Blurred Vision	☐
Neck Pain	☐	Diarrhea	☐
Visual Aura	☐	Confusion	☐

Daily Migraine Log

Date:

Migraine: Y   N

Sleep:	Time Asleep:	Total Hours:	Notes:
	Time Awake:	Quality: ☆☆☆☆☆	

		What I ate and drank	Medicines	How I feel
Breakfast	Time:			
Snack	Time:			
Lunch	Time:			
Snack	Time:			
Dinner	Time:			
Snack	Time:			

Exercise:

Time:	Description:	How I Felt:
Duration:		

Relaxation:

Time:	Description:	How I Felt:
Duration:		

Stress:

Time:	Description:	How I Felt:
Duration:		

Weather:

High Temp:	Atmospheric Pressure:	Notes:

Other:

Time Outside:	Screen Time:	Do you have your period:	Water Drank:

Headache:

0 1 2 3 4 5 6 7 8 9 10

Notes:

Head Location:

Time Onset:	Duration:
Medication:	Did it Help?:

Other Symptoms::

Nausea ☐	Nasal Congestion ☐
Vomiting ☐	Sensitivity to Smell ☐
Sensitivity to Light ☐	Ringing in Ears / Tinnitus ☐
Sensitivity to Noise ☐	Blurred Vision ☐
Neck Pain ☐	Diarrhea ☐
Visual Aura ☐	Confusion ☐

Daily Migraine Log

Sleep:	Time Asleep:	Total Hours:	Notes:
	Time Awake:	Quality: ☆ ☆ ☆ ☆ ☆	

		What I ate and drank	Medicines	How I feel
Breakfast	Time:			
Snack	Time:			
Lunch	Time:			
Snack	Time:			
Dinner	Time:			
Snack	Time:			

Exercise:	Time: Duration:	Description:	How I Felt:
Relaxation:	Time: Duration:	Description:	How I Felt:
Stress:	Time: Duration:	Description:	How I Felt:

Weather:

High Temp:	Atmospheric Pressure:	Notes:

Other:

Time Outside:	Screen Time:	Do you have your period:	Water Drank:

Headache:

0 1 2 3 4 5 6 7 8 9 10	Notes:
Head Location:	
Time Onset: / Duration:	
Medication: / Did it Help?:	

Other Symptoms::

Nausea	☐	Nasal Congestion	☐
Vomiting	☐	Sensitivity to Smell	☐
Sensitivity to Light	☐	Ringing in Ears / Tinnitus	☐
Sensitivity to Noise	☐	Blurred Vision	☐
Neck Pain	☐	Diarrhea	☐
Visual Aura	☐	Confusion	☐

Date:

Migraine: Y   N

Daily Migraine Log

Sleep:	Time Asleep:	Total Hours:	Notes:
	Time Awake:	Quality: ☆ ☆ ☆ ☆ ☆	

		What I ate and drank	Medicines	How I feel
Breakfast	Time:			
Snack	Time:			
Lunch	Time:			
Snack	Time:			
Dinner	Time:			
Snack	Time:			

Exercise:

Time:	Description:	How I Felt:
Duration:		

Relaxation:

Time:	Description:	How I Felt:
Duration:		

Stress:

Time:	Description:	How I Felt:
Duration:		

Weather:

High Temp:	Atmospheric Pressure:	Notes:

Other:

Time Outside:	Screen Time:	Do you have your period:	Water Drank:

Headache:

0 1 2 3 4 5 6 7 8 9 10	Notes:

Head Location:

Time Onset:	Duration:
Medication:	Did it Help?:

Other Symptoms::

Nausea	☐	Nasal Congestion	☐
Vomiting	☐	Sensitivity to Smell	☐
Sensitivity to Light	☐	Ringing in Ears / Tinnitus	☐
Sensitivity to Noise	☐	Blurred Vision	☐
Neck Pain	☐	Diarrhea	☐
Visual Aura	☐	Confusion	☐

Date:

Migraine: Y   N

Daily Migraine Log

Sleep:			
Time Asleep:	Total Hours:	Notes:	
Time Awake:	Quality: ☆☆☆☆☆		

		What I ate and drank	Medicines	How I feel
Breakfast	Time:			
Snack	Time:			
Lunch	Time:			
Snack	Time:			
Dinner	Time:			
Snack	Time:			

Exercise:

Time:	Description:	How I Felt:
Duration:		

Relaxation:

Time:	Description:	How I Felt:
Duration:		

Stress:

Time:	Description:	How I Felt:
Duration:		

Weather:

High Temp:	Atmospheric Pressure:	Notes:

Other:

Time Outside:	Screen Time:	Do you have your period:	Water Drank:

Headache:

0 1 2 3 4 5 6 7 8 9 10	Notes:

Head Location:

Time Onset:	Duration:
Medication:	Did it Help?:

Other Symptoms::

Nausea ☐	Nasal Congestion ☐
Vomiting ☐	Sensitivity to Smell ☐
Sensitivity to Light ☐	Ringing in Ears / Tinnitus ☐
Sensitivity to Noise ☐	Blurred Vision ☐
Neck Pain ☐	Diarrhea ☐
Visual Aura ☐	Confusion ☐

Daily Migraine Log

Sleep:	Time Asleep:	Total Hours:	Notes:
	Time Awake:	Quality: ☆ ☆ ☆ ☆ ☆	

		What I ate and drank	Medicines	How I feel
Breakfast	Time:			
Snack	Time:			
Lunch	Time:			
Snack	Time:			
Dinner	Time:			
Snack	Time:			

Exercise:

Time:	Description:	How I Felt:
Duration:		

Relaxation:

Time:	Description:	How I Felt:
Duration:		

Stress:

Time:	Description:	How I Felt:
Duration:		

Weather:

High Temp:	Atmospheric Pressure:	Notes:

☀ ⛅ ☁ ⛈ 🌧 🌧 🌨

Other:

Time Outside:	Screen Time:	Do you have your period:	Water Drank:

Headache:

0   1   2   3   4   5   6   7   8   9   10

Head Location:

Time Onset:	Duration:
Medication:	Did it Help?:

Notes:

Other Symptoms::

Nausea	☐	Nasal Congestion	☐
Vomiting	☐	Sensitivity to Smell	☐
Sensitivity to Light	☐	Ringing in Ears / Tinnitus	☐
Sensitivity to Noise	☐	Blurred Vision	☐
Neck Pain	☐	Diarrhea	☐
Visual Aura	☐	Confusion	☐

Daily Migraine Log

Date:

Migraine: Y   N

Sleep:	Time Asleep:	Total Hours:	Notes:
	Time Awake:	Quality: ☆ ☆ ☆ ☆ ☆	

		What I ate and drank	Medicines	How I feel
Breakfast	Time:			
Snack	Time:			
Lunch	Time:			
Snack	Time:			
Dinner	Time:			
Snack	Time:			

| Exercise: | Time: | Description: | How I Felt: |
| | Duration: | | |

| Relaxation: | Time: | Description: | How I Felt: |
| | Duration: | | |

| Stress: | Time: | Description: | How I Felt: |
| | Duration: | | |

Weather:

| High Temp: | Atmospheric Pressure: | Notes: |

Other:

| Time Outside: | Screen Time: | Do you have your period: | Water Drank: |

Headache:

0 1 2 3 4 5 6 7 8 9 10

Notes:

Head Location:

| Time Onset: | Duration: |
| Medication: | Did it Help?: |

Other Symptoms::

Nausea	☐	Nasal Congestion	☐
Vomiting	☐	Sensitivity to Smell	☐
Sensitivity to Light	☐	Ringing in Ears / Tinnitus	☐
Sensitivity to Noise	☐	Blurred Vision	☐
Neck Pain	☐	Diarrhea	☐
Visual Aura	☐	Confusion	☐

Daily Migraine Log

Date:

Migraine: Y   N

Sleep:	Time Asleep:	Total Hours:	Notes:
	Time Awake:	Quality: ☆ ☆ ☆ ☆ ☆	

		What I ate and drank	Medicines	How I feel
Breakfast	Time:			
Snack	Time:			
Lunch	Time:			
Snack	Time:			
Dinner	Time:			
Snack	Time:			

Exercise:	Time: Duration:	Description:	How I Felt:

Relaxation:	Time: Duration:	Description:	How I Felt:

Stress:	Time: Duration:	Description:	How I Felt:

Weather:

High Temp:	Atmospheric Pressure:	Notes:

Other:

Time Outside:	Screen Time:	Do you have your period:	Water Drank:

Headache:

0   1   2   3   4   5   6   7   8   9   10

Notes:

Head Location:

Time Onset:	Duration:
Medication:	Did it Help?:

Other Symptoms::

Nausea	☐	Nasal Congestion	☐
Vomiting	☐	Sensitivity to Smell	☐
Sensitivity to Light	☐	Ringing in Ears / Tinnitus	☐
Sensitivity to Noise	☐	Blurred Vision	☐
Neck Pain	☐	Diarrhea	☐
Visual Aura	☐	Confusion	☐

Made in United States
Orlando, FL
08 June 2023